breathe

breathe

The 4-week breathing
retraining plan to relieve
stress, anxiety and panic

MARY BIRCH

piatkus

PIATKUS

First published in Great Britain in 2019 by Piatkus

1 3 5 7 9 10 8 6 4 2

Text and illustrations copyright © 2019 Mary Birch

The moral right of the author has been asserted.

A CIP catalogue record for this book
is available from the British Library.

ISBN 978-0-349-42190-2

Cover design by Christabella Designs
Cover photograph courtesy of iStock
Typeset in Garamond Regular by Kirby Jones
Printed and bound in Great Britain by
Clays Ltd, Elcograf S.p.A

Papers used by Piatkus are from well-managed forests
and other responsible sources.

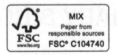

Piatkus
An imprint of
Little, Brown Book Group
Carmelite House
50 Victoria Embankment
London EC4Y 0DZ

An Hachette UK Company
www.hachette.co.uk

www.improvementzone.co.uk

Any advice in this book is general in nature and is not intended
as a substitute for medical advice and must not be relied upon as such.
For any healthcare advice, always consult a healthcare practitioner.

Pseudonyms have been used in this book and other details altered where
necessary to protect the identity and privacy of people mentioned.

To my husband, Chris,
and my children, Julia and Alex

Contents

Foreword

I was honoured to be approached by Mary Birch to write the foreword for this book. I first met Mary in 1999 when she made contact about undertaking the Buteyko Practitioner Training course.

In this book she shares her rich experience and provides significant practical information for the management of stress, anxiety and panic. The case studies will appeal to a wide range of readers as they give the human dimension to many common yet often overlooked consequences of incorrect breathing. Mary also provides readers with an insight into the important role of breathing retraining for other conditions, including asthma and sleep disorders, not to mention overall general health.

Mary's vast experience in nursing, health education and journalism in several countries provided her with a great platform for becoming a Breathing Educator. In addition, it immediately made her an invaluable asset for the Buteyko Institute of Breathing & Health (BIBH).

Along with the work in her own practice, Mary has led and been involved in numerous projects and initiatives on behalf of the BIBH over the years. These include:

- Developing and updating a theoretical written assessment system for accrediting new practitioners and upgrading existing practitioners.
- Designing, conducting, writing and distributing 'Sleep Apnoea – A Survey of Breathing Retraining'.
- Preparing applications for the research of breathing retraining with the Buteyko Institute Method for obstructive sleep apnoea.
- Providing information for private health insurers in relation to achieving rebate status for BIBH Practitioners.

I congratulate Mary for writing this book, and also for her contribution to disseminating significant information about the importance of correct breathing for improving health.

Paul O'Connell BSc, Dip Ed, MBA
Chief Executive Officer
Buteyko Institute of Breathing & Health

Introduction

If you are reading this book, the chances are that you or a loved one experiences stress, anxiety or panic attacks. It can be very scary when you feel anxious or panicky and have difficulty breathing.

Since 1999, I have taught breathing retraining classes for clients experiencing stress, anxiety and panic symptoms. I have witnessed their struggles, seen their tears and heard first hand their accounts of their attempts – sometimes for months, years or even decades – to overcome their symptoms, before they enrolled in the classes I teach.

My experience has taught me that of all the clients I have seen over the years, it is the people experiencing stress, anxiety and panic symptoms who are often the most isolated and despondent. They are sometimes advised to 'relax', 'take this medicine', 'take deep breaths' or 'stop over-analysing and you'll be fine'. But despite this well-intended advice, they are far from fine.

Clients who have successfully conquered anxiety and panic by improving their breathing pattern have urged me to write this book, because information on effective breathing retraining techniques – such as the ones I teach – is not readily available. My objective in writing this book is to redress this situation and to offer an effective, positive, realistic – and powerful – way to gain relief. I don't use the word 'powerful' lightly: I have witnessed the changes in my clients numerous times over the years.

Professor Konstantin Buteyko, the doctor who developed the breathing retraining method on which many of the exercises in this book are based, contended that over-breathing is not just a symptom of, but in fact the cause of, a wide range of illnesses, ranging from cardiac problems to breathing disorders.[1]

In fact, over-breathing could be said to be *the* major epidemic of modern living, yet it is largely unrecognised, misunderstood or often ignored. And, as you will discover while you read this book, over-breathing is responsible for numerous physical, emotional and psychological conditions, and can adversely affect sleep, mood and quality of life.

I have found that the majority of my clients experiencing stress, anxiety and panic are over-breathing, sometimes significantly. Generally, they are not aware that they are over-breathing, or that this is linked to their symptoms. Returning breathing to the normal level has an enormous impact on reducing or eliminating symptoms, and restoring a sense of calm.

Since I started teaching breathing retraining, I have been privileged to witness clients who had been experiencing stress, anxiety and panic symptoms transform their health and wellbeing, and regain their joie de vivre, without needing any extra medication and with no side effects. I am saddened by some of the stories from my clients who have struggled with anxiety, panic attacks, sleep and stress issues for years, when something as simple as breathing retraining could have provided relief. In 2015, I wrote an article on the subject of hyperventilation and breathing retraining in anxiety and panic disorders, which was published in the *Australian Nursing and Midwifery Journal*.[2] Following its publication, it was very gratifying to receive reports via other breathing retraining practitioners in Australia that members of the public who had read the article had benefited significantly just from following some of the basic information I provided in it, such as gentle nose-breathing.

Most people will begin to feel an improvement in their symptoms within a week of implementing the strategies I teach, sometimes even within a few days. But I recommend a minimum four-week breathing retraining program for a reason: the body has to adjust to the new and improved breathing pattern, and this improved breathing pattern needs to become automatic, so that the person does not revert to a disordered breathing pattern and chronic over-breathing in times of stress.

Part 1 of this book provides an explanation of the link between over-breathing and stress, anxiety and panic symptoms. Part 2 contains the four-week program with weekly guidelines to help people experiencing these issues to improve their breathing pattern and gain long-term relief.

The stories and people mentioned throughout this book are based on real events and real clients (or composites of real clients) but the names and any identifying details have been changed to protect the identities of the individuals. I hope these stories will strike a chord with people who are struggling with stress, anxiety and panic symptoms, and who may be feeling isolated, and give them hope that they are not alone and that their symptoms can be alleviated.

Conventional wisdom suggests that it takes three weeks to change a habit. Breathing is a habit that is *very* instinctive, and therefore, changing and improving breathing takes time. Added to this, some people with stress, anxiety and panic symptoms may be sensitive to the changes in body chemistry (even within the normal ranges) that may be part of breathing retraining. Improving something as automatic as breathing pattern requires time, effort, understanding and patience. Accordingly, there is a need to take things very slowly initially, as explained in Part 1 of this book.

For those who would like to delve into the scientific evidence, a comprehensive reference list and bibliography are provided.

Important advice

I recommend that you read the chapters in Part 1 of this book first, so that you can gain a clear understanding of how your breathing pattern is linked to stress, anxiety and panic symptoms, and of what to expect during breathing retraining. This will help you to understand the objectives you are trying to achieve in terms of improving your breathing pattern in Part 2.

However eager you are to get started, please don't be tempted to try the breathing retraining strategies without reading Part 1. I caution people to go slowly initially and take it step by step, because attempting to go too fast may *trigger* anxiety and panic symptoms in some people.

The strategies and recommendations provided in this book are aimed specifically at adults experiencing stress, anxiety and panic. This advice may not be appropriate or adequate for people suffering from asthma or other conditions. If you have asthma,

I recommend that you find an accredited practitioner. For further advice, please see Appendix 1. If you are pregnant or think you may become pregnant, or if you have a current breathing condition or any other medical condition, I recommend that you follow your doctor's advice before starting any of the breathing retraining exercises contained in this book. Also, do not reduce or cease any medication without the guidance of your doctor.

As there are several medical conditions that may be associated with anxiety and panic symptoms, I advise anyone with these symptoms to consult their doctor.

Mary Birch
Melbourne, Australia
2019

PART 1

KNOWLEDGE
IS POWER

CHAPTER 1

The role of breathing in stress, anxiety and panic

'So it's not all in my head?'

Jonathan is a pleasant, easygoing man who attended my breathing retraining practice many years ago. Outwardly happy and content with his life, with interesting hobbies and a very supportive family, Jonathan looked the picture of health. But he had experienced anxiety and panic attacks for more than a decade. Life had become a real struggle and he couldn't seem to find a way through.

When I assessed Jonathan's pulse, I noticed that it was extremely irregular. He smiled when I mentioned this to him and said that he was aware of it, that it had been like that for years and had been thoroughly investigated. In fact, Jonathan had undergone several investigations into his heart and other body systems over the years, but nothing had ever been found to account for his irregular pulse or for his anxiety and panic attacks.

I explained to Jonathan that his breathing pattern had become disordered and he was over-breathing. This 'faulty' breathing pattern had become a habit and might be the cause of some of his symptoms.

'So I'm not going crazy!' he responded – then he burst into tears. It was a huge relief for him to discover that his symptoms could be improved just by retraining his breathing.

To his delight, Jonathan began to see an improvement in many of his symptoms during the breathing retraining course. Two weeks after the course, he returned to the breathing centre for a follow-up review with a story to tell.

'You'll never guess what's happened!' he said. 'My pulse is regular and I haven't had a panic attack since I did the course.'

This was really heartening news from someone who had almost given up on finding a way to get rid of his symptoms, and who, just three weeks earlier, had begun to think that he was becoming mentally unstable. It was my turn to have tears in my eyes.

Do you experience recurring anxiety? Does the thought of making a simple decision leave you almost paralysed with fear? Do you worry about things that may never happen? Maybe you don't sleep well and feel exhausted most of the time? Outwardly it may look as if you have it all, but inwardly you feel alone, isolated and that nobody really understands you.*

It's strange that anxiety is so common, yet is so rarely discussed either in the workplace or in social situations. According to

---

* If you need immediate help in coping with anxiety, panic or depression, please see the Resources section at the end of this book for links to organisations that offer support.

Mind, a registered UK charity, a 2016 survey estimates that 5.9% of adults in England experience generalised anxiety disorder, 2.4% experience phobias, 1.3% experience obsessive-compulsive disorder, 0.6% experience panic disorder and 7.8% experience mixed anxiety and depression. All of these disorders were found to be more prevalent in women than in men.[1]

If you suffer stress, anxiety or panic symptoms, you might have tried a few different approaches in an attempt to free yourself from them, like Jonathan in the story. Yet despite your best efforts, those annoying, debilitating – and sometimes frightening – symptoms are still present. You might not even have considered that how you breathe may be triggering, let alone fuelling or sustaining, your symptoms. However, the bottom line is that if you aren't breathing correctly, this is almost certainly affecting your mood and causing physical and psychological symptoms.

Here is a quick breathing assessment:

- Are you mouth-breathing – either chronically or from time to time?
- Do you feel short of breath when exercising or when you are anxious or panicky?
- Do you feel as if you are shallow-breathing at times?
- Even when it's nowhere near bedtime, do you sigh or yawn excessively?
- Do you have a hunger for air, or sometimes feel as if you can never get enough air?

If you answered yes to any of these questions, it is highly likely that you are over-breathing and you would benefit from breathing retraining.

> Over-breathing – or 'hyperventilation' to use
> the medical term – is the plague of modern
> life and may affect up to 25 per cent of the
> population. Yet many people may not be aware
> that they are over-breathing, and may continue
> to struggle with high stress levels, anxiety
> and/or panic attacks for months or years.

Over-breathing is part of a breathing pattern that can be called 'dysfunctional' or disordered. A dysfunctional breathing pattern means that a person is not breathing within the normal breathing ranges. And, as we have seen in Jonathan's story, **over-breathing** is one of the key components of ongoing stress, anxiety and panic symptoms. The link between over-breathing and stress, anxiety and panic is well established and is supported by an abundance of scientific evidence.[2]

But why are we over-breathing? The short answer is: a combination of myth, habit and evolution. The stresses of modern living, combined with the myths surrounding the benefits of deep breathing, which started in the twentieth century, have taken their toll.

Far from being good for us, as most people assume, deliberate deep breathing can develop into an unhealthy habit of over-breathing. ('Over-breathing' and 'hyperventilation' mean exactly the same thing. In this book, I prefer to use the term 'over-breathing' rather than the medical term 'hyperventilation'. This is because most people associate hyperventilation with obviously loud, noisy, deep or rapid breathing, or puffing up the chest – and that is not the case in the vast majority of those who are hyperventilating.) So instead of a deep breath, take a long, slow, *gentle* breath. Reducing stress, anxiety and panic symptoms just by improving the way you breathe is not only possible, it is literally under your control.

Deep breathing, normal breathing, over-breathing

First, let us take a look at what constitutes normal breathing. Sometimes when I ask my clients to take a normal breath, they look at me in surprise and say, 'I don't know what a normal breath is any more.'

Normal breathing, as depicted in the left-hand column of Table 1.1 overleaf, is effortless, regular, gentle and inaudible (unless exercising or working strenuously) and, of course, comfortable. Normal breathing means we are able to nose-breathe comfortably at rest (while seated or sleeping) or while walking around.

Our breathing and our heart rates are subject to change throughout the day (and night) and they usually work in unison. When we feel stressed or anxious, or when we have a fever, our heart and breathing rates increase; conversely, when we are relaxed, they decrease.

'Over-breathing' can be defined as breathing too fast or too deeply, or a combination of both. Breathing in this manner does not allow an adequate exchange of gases in the body, so the balance of gases is disturbed, often leading to numerous physical and/or psychological symptoms, depending on the degree of over-breathing.

TABLE 1.1: CONTRASTING NORMAL BREATHING AND OVER-BREATHING IN ADULTS	
NORMAL BREATHING	**OVER-BREATHING**
Effortless	Struggling for air, cannot take a deep enough breath, air hunger, shortness of breath, breathlessness.
Regular rhythm	Erratic or irregular breathing pattern, episodes of shallow breathing, intermittent deep breaths. Daytime apnoeas or pauses in breathing pattern, often resuming breathing with a gasp.
Gentle nose-breathing at rest and when walking	Mouth-breathing at rest or when walking, deep breathing at rest or when walking.
Comfortable nasal breathing	Blocked nose, increased mucus, dry mouth, post-nasal drip (mucus drip at the back of the nose).
Inaudible breathing at rest	Noisy or audible breathing at rest, sighing or yawning excessively, gasping for air, throat-clearing or tickly cough evident, taking audible or deeper breaths when speaking.
Refreshing sleep	Increased waking, poor or unrefreshing sleep, waking with a headache, waking with a dry mouth, needing water by the bedside.
Posture upright, shoulders back and relaxed	Slumped posture, head thrust forwards, shoulders raised and forwards, tension in neck, jaw or shoulders.
Breathing from the diaphragm	Breathing from upper chest (thoracic breathing), upper chest expansion obvious on inhalation.
A breathing rate of 8–14 breaths/min.	Increased breathing rate at rest – though not always evident if breathing deeply or mouth-breathing.
Pulse rate regular, within normal range	Increased pulse rate, palpitations, irregular pulse.
Minute volume: 4–6L/min.	Minute volume in excess of 6L/min.
End-tidal carbon dioxide levels within normal range	Decreased end-tidal carbon dioxide levels.

Breathing more deeply while exercising or when engaged in some strenuous physical activity (e.g. digging the garden, playing sports or running for a train) is perfectly normal and is to be expected. During vigorous activities we need more oxygen, and therefore we need to breathe faster and more deeply. However, *deliberate* deep breathing – whether from the chest or from the diaphragm – is not appropriate and may lead to over-breathing.

But how do we know when someone is over-breathing? One of the objective measures used is to assess carbon dioxide levels. Carbon dioxide is not just a waste gas, as we may have been led to believe – a certain level of this gas in the body is essential for many processes. It is produced during our cells' energy production, and as we breathe out it is exhaled. Over-breathing leads to excessive loss of carbon dioxide and it is this reduction in carbon dioxide levels that leads to adverse symptoms.

I use a scientific instrument called a capnometer or capnograph to assess and monitor the breathing patterns of my clients.[3] This instrument measures the 'end-tidal' carbon dioxide levels, that is, the end of the stream of air as we breathe out. End-tidal carbon dioxide ($ETCO_2$) levels are reduced in people who are over-breathing. As the volume of air we breathe (called the 'minute volume') is increased in over-breathing, the amount of carbon dioxide we exhale is also increased, leading to reduced carbon dioxide levels.

One study found that end-tidal carbon dioxide levels in patients experiencing anxiety were as low as those in patients with panic disorder.[4] In effect, this suggests that people with anxiety – and who do not experience panic attacks – may over-breathe as much as people experiencing panic disorder.

Although the normal breathing pattern shown in Table 1.1 seems fairly obvious, we often lack awareness of what our breathing pattern is really like. In fact, in the majority of cases the over-breathing pattern may not be obvious to the person themselves or even to their doctor. Breathing is so instinctive that we are mostly unaware of it until we develop obvious symptoms such as shortness of breath or tightness or pain in the chest.

In practice, I have found that the vast majority of clients experiencing stress, anxiety and panic symptoms over-breathe on a regular basis. In addition, I have found that most people experiencing these conditions have a very irregular or erratic breathing pattern. However, they are generally not aware of this pattern. They may say, 'I breathe too shallowly' or 'I feel short of breath' or 'I can never get enough air'.

As you will discover from this book, habitual or chronic over-breathing is a significant trigger for – and in many cases may be the fundamental cause of – not only increased stress levels and anxiety and panic symptoms, but also several other apparently unrelated symptoms.

Depending on the degree of over-breathing, numerous signs and symptoms may also be present. For example, people who over-breathe may have an irregular breathing pattern, experience periods of shallow breathing, may sigh frequently, or their breathing may be audible to others, but they may not be aware of it. Symptoms such as a 'hunger for air' or not being able to take adequately deep breaths may also be present. Also, people who are over-breathing may feel short of breath and experience difficulty in breathing, or be unable to exercise comfortably.

Surprisingly, the number of breaths per minute may not be increased in over-breathing. If someone is taking deeper breaths, frequently sighing or yawning, or mouth-breathing, the number of breaths per minute may remain within the normal range.

Quite often (but not inevitably) the person who is over-breathing may be mouth-breathing, sometimes without realising that this is happening. Due to constant mouth-breathing they may have a dry mouth, especially on waking, because they have been mouth-breathing throughout the night. In addition, sleep may be unrefreshing or they may have insomnia. During the day, their nose may tend to block and they may have increased mucus, sinus issues or an occasional dry, tickly cough.

Headaches, fatigue and palpitations are also fairly common with over-breathing. Occasionally, when the over-breathing is severe, it may cause tingling in the hands or feet or around the lips.

Many of my clients report that they are shallow-breathing, and therefore they conclude that they cannot be over-breathing. It is quite natural to suspect that we are not breathing enough air because of shallow breathing, whereas the opposite is most likely true: shallow-breathing is a sign of a disordered breathing pattern and is a characteristic of *over*-breathing. Shallow-breathing is more likely to be due to an increased volume of air inhaled. When this happens, it is thought that there is so much air already in the lungs that the person has difficulty inhaling a normal volume of air with the next breath, due to the increased residual air already in the lungs.

Depending on stress levels and breathing habits, over-breathing may be either chronic or intermittent. In both cases, improving the breathing pattern through breathing retraining will lead to a significant improvement in symptoms.

What is breathing retraining?

The method of breathing retraining I teach is an educational program called the Buteyko method, which incorporates a broad range of specific strategies, breathing exercises and techniques aimed at normalising a disordered breathing pattern. As this is not an exercise program, there is no strenuous physical activity involved. All of the breathing retraining exercises can be done while seated or standing. In the short term, the improvement in breathing leads to a reduction in symptoms. Total elimination of symptoms takes longer, as the new and improved breathing pattern needs to become automatic. Although the exercises are easy, it is not a quick fix and takes time, effort and patience.

A book cannot provide the full range of practices and guidance that a Buteyko breathing retraining course run by an accredited practitioner can provide. Therefore, I have adapted some of the strategies so that the average person experiencing stress, anxiety or panic can follow the program at their own pace week by week.

In this book you will learn how to recognise over-breathing. You will also have an opportunity to assess your breathing pattern using a questionnaire. You will discover how over-breathing is linked to stress, anxiety and panic symptoms, and you may be shocked to find that deep breathing is not as good for us as we have been led to believe.

If you are experiencing high stress levels, persistent anxiety or panic attacks, then the good news is that improving your breathing pattern will help you to break free from the over-breathing habit. It will take a little of your time every day for a minimum of four weeks, but you will be rewarded for your efforts with a significant improvement in your health and quality of life.

When your breathing pattern is normalised, the anxiety and panic symptoms will become a thing of the past and your ability to adapt to stress will also improve. And like my client Jonathan, once you see that you are improving, your motivation to improve will increase, and you will find that there is a light at the end of the stress, anxiety or panic attacks tunnel.

'Knowledge is power' is my mantra, and in this book you will find the knowledge to take responsibility for your health, retrain your breathing pattern and heal yourself.

CHAPTER 2

The over-breathing cycle

How over-breathing fuels anxiety symptoms

Emily, a pleasant woman in her sixties, attended the breathing centre with her husband for help with panic attacks, which had begun following surgery several months before. After investigation, Emily's doctor had reassured her that there were no physical reasons for her symptoms. Emily and her husband were very concerned. Nothing Emily tried had helped, and the panic attacks, which were occurring almost daily, were having an impact on the couple's quality of life. Emily was reluctant to leave their home, or do anything on her own, in case a panic attack started.

A friend suggested breathing retraining, so Emily's husband encouraged her to enrol in a course. I observed that Emily had signs of over-breathing, such as mouth-breathing and excessive sighing and yawning. She told me her sleep was also affected and she kept waking at night. I explained that the stress of surgery may have affected Emily's breathing pattern, causing her to over-breathe and triggering the panic attacks. Even though Emily had made a good recovery from the surgery, the over-breathing habit continued.

Emily gradually improved during the breathing retraining course, she was sleeping better and the panic attacks diminished. When Emily and her husband returned for a follow-up review two weeks later, they both looked much happier. Emily said she was still a little anxious at times but the panic attacks had stopped.

One month later I was surprised to get a call from Emily's husband. Emily was doing fine, he reported, and not having the panic attacks. Best of all, they had booked an overseas holiday – the first in a long time.

We all experience high anxiety levels at some point in our lives; anxiety is part of being human and is a normal emotion that is key to our survival. For some people, prolonged and excessive anxiety casts a shadow that may significantly affect their day-to-day life or may even prevent them from doing the things they need to do. But why would the anxiety persist if the danger is past, or if there is no actual threat?

Are your survival instincts set on high alert?

Life is not enjoyable when we are anxious. Stress, anxiety, fear and worry may have a huge impact on our ability to cope with daily living. At its extreme, anxiety can prevent us from doing things such as going out, meeting people, having a relationship, socialising, changing careers, and even earning a living. When we are anxious all the time we can't relax, and everything becomes a challenge. The survival instinct, which has protected us throughout our evolution, has now become over-protective and is set on high alert; it is out of proportion to the degree of risk or danger. Increased breathing is normal when there is danger; it allows us to run or fight. But when breathing is constantly increased and there is no potential or actual danger, we have developed an unhealthy habit: over-breathing.

The over-breathing habit

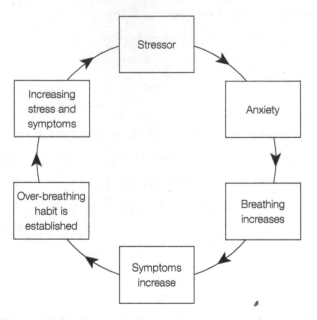

Figure 2.1: Stress, anxiety and the over-breathing cycle

The connection between stress, anxiety, panic and over-breathing is well documented, but most people are not aware that it is the *over-breathing* habit that may be helping to fuel or sustain ongoing stress, anxiety and panic symptoms.[1] When we are exposed to stressors – that is, when we feel stressed or anxious –

our breathing pattern changes. (Stressors are situations or events that cause us to feel stressed and provoke a stress response in the body.) We may breathe more deeply, or our breathing rate may increase. In some people there may be a combination of deeper breathing *and* an increased breathing rate. This is when stress and anxiety can lead to the development of the over-breathing habit, as depicted in Figure 2.1. Breathing three or four times the normal volume of air – which occurs in over-breathing – is physically taxing and places an additional strain on the body. It also acts as an unconscious stressor, increasing physical and psychological symptoms, leading to sleep issues and fatigue.

While stress may have triggered the initial anxiety and panic symptoms, it is the over-breathing habit that then takes centre stage and sustains and fuels the symptoms. Long after the stressful period has ended, over-breathing continues to trigger or cause anxiety or panic symptoms.

I have seen clients who developed anxiety and panic symptoms following physical stressors such as a prolonged lack of refreshing sleep, major illness or surgery, trauma or accidents. Psychological stressors, including work-related pressures, bullying, job loss, relationship issues, divorce or bereavement, can also cause the stress response to activate and the breathing pattern to change.

The key to understanding our increasing stress levels lies in our evolutionary past. We survived and succeeded as a species simply because we had the capacity to become anxious, breathe more deeply, and either run away or fight. We escaped danger and lived long enough to procreate and pass on those survival instincts to our children.

ANXIETY SIGNS AND SYMPTOMS

- Worry, rumination (constantly going over uncomfortable or hypothetical situations in our minds)
- Increased heart rate, palpitations
- Muscle tension
- Tightness in chest, chest pain
- Difficulty in breathing, shortness of breath
- Sleep problems
- Appetite changes
- Mood changes
- Irritability
- Decreased confidence
- Sweating
- Shaking
- Headache, light-headedness
- Twitching or tics
- Tingling sensations in fingers or extremities

But nowadays we do not become anxious for short periods and afterwards relax and recuperate as we did when we were hunter-gatherers. Many of us are feeling chronically stressed and anxious – and are therefore over-breathing – most of the time. It's normal to feel stressed or anxious when we are under threat or when we fear something unpleasant, dangerous or harmful may occur. But when the danger has passed and we continue to over-breathe, the anxiety persists as if we were still under threat and we experience physical and psychological symptoms as shown in the list of Anxiety Signs and Symptoms. These symptoms are very real and are not imaginary, as some people might suppose. Many of these signs and symptoms are directly associated with over-breathing, e.g. an increased heart rate, palpitations, sweating, shaking, twitching, difficulty in breathing and shortness of breath.

Putting anxiety into perspective

Could you imagine a world without anxiety? Where everyone is always happy and nothing is too much trouble? Where we always wake up in the morning with a smile on our face and go to bed at night feeling relaxed, content and at peace? Where the words 'no worries' would literally mean just that? It sounds like a fictitious place: Utopia.

The truth is, if there were no anxiety we could not survive. We would not bother to go to work because we would not see the need to earn an income. We would not need to go looking for food because we would have no anxiety about when or where our next meal was coming from, and we would most likely starve as a result. We would take risks and probably fall off a cliff or walk in front of a car – assuming, of course, that someone bothered to design and build a car, or even learn to drive!

Anxiety is *not* a weakness as some people may believe. Anxiety has protected us and kept us safe through the centuries as we evolved, often in hostile environments, to become the dominant species on this planet. A certain amount of anxiety can help us perform better, remain alert and even excel at what we do. Those butterflies in the stomach generally settle down as we progress with our presentation or come to grips with that daunting exam, as the adrenaline rush that occurs as part of the stress response also settles down.

Don't suffer in silence

While anxiety is normal and is to be expected in some situations, persistent and severe anxiety may affect our health and our quality of life, and may lead to depression. Therefore, it's important not to allow the anxiety to continue, especially if it is affecting sleep or daily activities, and to seek help. Seeing your doctor for guidance is important. Anxiety is one of the most common conditions seen in general practice, and is something that most family physicians see on a daily basis. While there are anxiety screening tools and questionnaires available online, these do not replace the need to consult your doctor.

Counselling, cognitive behavioural therapy and/or medication are generally the health management strategies of choice for anxiety and panic symptoms. Other approaches may include relaxation techniques, lifestyle adjustments (such as attention to diet, exercise and sleep), and stress management techniques. I would add breathing retraining to this list.

However daunting all this may sound, bear in mind that you are a *survivor*. Give yourself credit for having survived.

CHAPTER 3

Panic and over-breathing

Anxiety, adrenaline and panic

'You are my last hope.'

The young man seated before me seemed exhausted, ill at ease and defeated. Slumped, pale, and apparently at a low ebb, Josh explained that stress and anxiety had plagued his life for many years, but now he had reached rock bottom. Lacking in confidence, not sleeping well and no longer able to work or study, he had started having panic attacks. He said he felt really exhausted and just couldn't concentrate. He sighed and yawned constantly as he explained his concerns.

My young client had consulted his doctor and tried numerous therapies without success, so it seemed I was his last, desperate, hope. But he was not optimistic and appeared quite sceptical as to whether I could really help him.

I assessed Josh's breathing pattern using a capnometer. The results were displayed on a computer screen and Josh was able to see his breathing pattern and his heart and breathing rates in graph form, along with the levels of end-tidal carbon dioxide.

Josh's assessment showed a very irregular breathing pattern. Every few breaths he would sigh as he exhaled, which showed up as a jagged downward line on his out-breath. In addition, his breathing rate was quite fast, at 20 breaths per minute. The optimal breathing range for a young adult is 8–14 breaths per minute. Josh's end-tidal carbon dioxide levels were reduced, and indicated that he was moderately over-breathing.

Josh continued to sigh and yawn throughout the first few sessions of his breathing retraining course, but gradually his breathing pattern settled down and he appeared noticeably calmer and at ease. He even began to smile, engage in conversation and make jokes, which was great to see.

As I suggested, Josh continued with the daily breathing retraining exercises and when we repeated his breathing assessment a couple of weeks later, his breathing pattern had improved significantly and his panic attacks had ceased. His breathing had become regular, the sighing respiration was gone, and the number of breaths per minute was a very normal 12. His end-tidal carbon dioxide levels were now in the normal to optimal range. Josh's sleep had also improved and he was scoring himself 8 out of 10 on sleep quality, whereas before the course he had scored himself 3 out of 10. The fatigue had also improved and he was planning to return to the gym and start jogging on a daily basis to improve his fitness level.

I explained to Josh that he would need to continue with the breathing exercises for a few weeks longer in order to reinforce his improved breathing pattern and ensure that it remained within the normal range even if under stress. After such a significant improvement, Josh was happy to continue the exercises for a few weeks; he was optimistic and looking forward to returning to work and study, and getting on with his life.

Panic disorder is a condition where repeated, unexpected attacks of intense fear or panic attacks occur. Just as the panic attack starts, there is a feeling of dread, a feeling of not being able to breathe, a fear of becoming extremely embarrassed or thinking that everyone is noticing. Panic attacks may happen out of the blue, sometimes with no known cause, or they may be related to severe anxiety.

Panic attacks can be devastating and draining, and can be the bane of some people's lives. They can lead to increased stress, poor health, sleep issues, loss of confidence and feelings of isolation. People experiencing panic attacks are inevitably stressed and anxious, and are also almost inevitably over-breathing, either intermittently or chronically. If you experience anxiety or panic attacks, improving your breathing pattern is key to becoming well.

There are several theories why panic attacks occur and, for the most part, these are based on dysfunctional or disordered breathing patterns. There is a hyperventilation-based theory of panic disorder, which has existed for decades. In this theory, people with panic disorder are thought to be chronically over-breathing and, as a result, their carbon dioxide levels are constantly reduced. These low carbon dioxide levels may result in increased anxiety and poor health. In effect, when people who are chronically over-breathing become stressed, they over-breathe even more, their carbon dioxide levels drop even further, and the result is a panic attack.

Breathing faster, taking deeper breaths,
yawning and sighing are some of the ways
to quickly reduce those carbon dioxide levels
back to a more comfortable level – even if
that level is lower than normal. So in effect
the over-breathing pattern is sustained
through a habit of over-breathing.

In fact, evidence suggesting over-breathing has been found in several studies of panic disorder.[1] Some studies have shown significantly lower baseline end-tidal carbon dioxide levels among people with panic disorder than in people with generalised anxiety disorder or among healthy controls.[2]

Correct levels of carbon dioxide in the body are very important for certain key functions, and these levels are monitored and regulated by the breathing or respiratory centre, which is located at the base of the brain. We all have a range of carbon dioxide levels we are accustomed to, i.e. a 'threshold' for carbon dioxide levels. People who chronically over-breathe may become accustomed to reduced carbon dioxide levels – which means the over-breathing pattern is reinforced. In addition, studies suggest that the breathing pattern in people with panic disorder may be irregular and that 'respiratory variability', or a disordered breathing pattern, may make some people more vulnerable to panic attacks.[3] So when people who are already continuously over-breathing become stressed, they may respond by breathing even more deeply or faster. This may be enough to trigger a panic attack due to very low carbon dioxide levels and activation of the fight-or-flight response, including the adrenaline rush that accompanies panic attacks.

In some people, the respiratory centre takes action when it finds that we are coming close to or have moved beyond the upper level of carbon dioxide that we are accustomed to. Breathing faster, taking deeper breaths, yawning and sighing are some of the ways to quickly reduce carbon dioxide to a comfortable level – even if that level is lower than normal.

Many of my clients with panic attacks can attest to the fact that they had experienced anxiety for some time before the panic attacks began. Some clients report that they've always been anxious, even as a child. Most clients say that they had panic symptoms for at least six months before they attended breathing retraining classes. Sadly, some of my clients say they have had the condition for years or even decades.

I have found that people with panic disorder are often generally unwell. They may experience increased or recurring anxiety between panic attacks and mostly they do not sleep well. In fact, panic disorder is actually considered a type of anxiety disorder.[4] There may be a cycle of chronic over-breathing, which contributes to the anxiety and panic symptoms, where one leads to the other and the person remains in poor health.[5] This may create a self-perpetuating mechanism in some people where the over-breathing and panic attacks continue to occur and link into each other.

When someone is having a panic attack, their heart rate increases, as does their breathing. However, because of the difficulty of capturing or monitoring real-life panic attacks either before or during an attack, the actual incidence of over-breathing *during* a panic attack is not known with any degree of certainty, although the association between over-breathing and panic disorder has been well documented in medical literature.[6]

As the fight-or-flight response is activated during a panic attack, and breathing is increased as a result of this response, it may be argued that *all* panic attacks involve over-breathing, either before or during the attack.

It seems that not all panic attacks occur for the same reasons; several different theories – most based on dysfunctional or disordered breathing – have been put forward. The hyperventilation-based theory mentioned above is one. Another hypothesis is that some people with panic disorder may have a false suffocation alarm, which triggers their panic attacks.[7] This means that a 'suffocation monitor' in the brain can misfire and lead to panic symptoms when levels of carbon dioxide *increase* – which is the exact opposite to the hyperventilation-based theory.

Most people who have experienced a panic attack will recognise and identify with some of the symptoms in Table 3.1 (on page 36). These symptoms may be very frightening, and the day-to-day effects on people experiencing panic disorder can be profound. Panic symptoms are often challenging and, unsurprisingly, they can have a huge impact on quality of life, sleep, confidence and general health. In some instances the person may become depressed or they may develop a dependency on alcohol or drugs as they struggle to overcome their symptoms. Unfortunately, symptoms may increase over time.

What happens during a panic attack?

A panic attack sets in train a cascade of physical, hormonal and emotional events in the body, as set out in Table 3.1. Although everything may seem to happen at once, there are certain stages through which a person may progress while having a panic attack. Not everyone will have exactly the same sequence of events or the same symptoms or progression. Everyone is different, but there are similarities.

The fight-or-flight response is activated early on in a panic attack. This is a primitive – and protective – survival mechanism, controlled by the autonomic nervous system.[8] In addition, the limbic system contains structures deep in the brain that evolved in early mammals and are related to anxiety, fear, anger, memory and survival. These systems evolved even before we had to either fight the woolly mammoth (or other predators) or run away, and this response still enables us to run or fight, and, most importantly, to survive. We still need – and use – these survival mechanisms today, if we sense we are in danger.

Just as the panic attack starts, there may be a feeling of dread, a feeling that something is not right, and this may be followed by a pounding heart, palpitations and chest tightness. Breathing deepens, and the person begins to feel short of breath or has difficulty in breathing, and they may develop chest pain. They may begin trembling and sweating, and they may experience tingling in the fingers, toes or even the face.

As the attack progresses, the person may begin to feel nauseated or develop a feeling of unreality. They may also feel faint and dizzy. The person may also become very embarrassed when they feel a panic attack coming on, as they may think that everyone must be aware of what is happening. The urge to escape becomes paramount, and the person is convinced that if they cannot escape in time, they may lose control, faint or even die. The reduction in carbon dioxide levels during a panic attack leads to spasms or narrowing of the blood vessels to the brain, which also reduces oxygen to the brain.[9, 10]

In addition, glucose, which is the fuel for brain cells, may be reduced, as stores of glucose in the liver are used up to prepare the person to fight or flee. As a result, low blood sugar levels (hypoglycaemia) may also cause the person to feel sweaty, shaky or light-headed. Not infrequently, people are taken to an emergency department for investigation when they have a panic attack, as the whole experience may be similar to a heart attack and is very frightening.[11]

These are extremely unpleasant symptoms that some people experience on a regular basis, sometimes for years. Small wonder, then, that some people may start to question if they are doing something physically, mentally or emotionally to trigger the panic attacks. I like to reassure people that they are not doing anything consciously to trigger the attacks. They are most likely not even aware of the over-breathing, because it has become a habit. The over-breathing habit, combined with increasing stress levels, is triggering their panic. And, like most habits, over-breathing can be changed.

As you can see from Table 3.1 below, several organs and systems in the body are affected during the fight-or-flight response. These include: the heart and blood vessels; the lungs and respiratory system; the stomach, pancreas and gastro-intestinal system; the liver; the brain and nervous system; the muscles; and hormones such as cortisol, adrenaline and insulin.

TABLE 3.1: WHAT ACTUALLY HAPPENS DURING A PANIC ATTACK?		
SIGNS AND SYMPTOMS	WHY?	RELATED ISSUES/ CAUSES
A feeling of dread; a feeling that something is not right.	We are on high alert: the sympathetic nervous system is activated and the fight-or-flight response kicks into action.	This is the body's natural reaction to stress or to a perceived threat.

TABLE 3.1: WHAT ACTUALLY HAPPENS DURING A PANIC ATTACK?		
SIGNS AND SYMPTOMS	WHY?	RELATED ISSUES/ CAUSES
A pounding heart, palpitations	Cardiac output is increased. Adrenaline and noradrenaline, the fight-or-flight hormones, are released, increasing the heart rate and the blood pressure to get us ready to fight or flee. Cortisol is also released within minutes.	Circulating blood flow increases. Blood is diverted to the large muscles of the arms and legs, giving us the extra oxygen to fight or flee. Increased cortisol means we will be able to fight or escape without feeling our injuries so much.
Breathing increases. Feeling short of breath or having difficulty breathing, chest tightness, chest pain.	Breathing increases due to an adrenaline rush, to allow us to fight or run.	Bronchioles – small air tubes – dilate to allow more air in and out of the lungs. We may be breathing so fast or so deeply we just cannot get any more air in.
Pupils dilate and senses sharpen.	We need to be able to remain alert and keep a sharp lookout to escape.	Hypervigilance will help us to survive.
Sweating	Keeps us cool to allow us to fight or flee.	May also be associated with low blood sugar levels. Glucose stores from the liver are released for extra energy requirements.
Nausea	Blood is being diverted from the stomach to the large muscles of the arms and legs to allow us to fight or run.	Digestion is decreased; the most important thing right now is to fight or flee. More oxygen is needed in the arms and legs.
Trembling	The nervous system is now involved, getting ready to go. Trembling may also be associated with low blood sugar levels (hypoglycaemia).	Insulin is produced to use the glucose stores from the liver in an effort to sustain energy increases (muscles, heart and breathing rates).

TABLE 3.1: WHAT ACTUALLY HAPPENS DURING A PANIC ATTACK?		
SIGNS AND SYMPTOMS	WHY?	RELATED ISSUES/ CAUSES
Tingling in extremities	Carbon dioxide levels are becoming very low due to over-breathing.	The nervous system has become sensitive and irritated.
Feeling dizzy or faint	The brain needs oxygen, but reduced carbon dioxide levels due to over-breathing prevent effective release of oxygen from red blood cells. This is called the Bohr effect.	Blood circulation to the brain is becoming impaired due to spasms in blood vessels caused by lowered carbon dioxide levels. Blood sugar levels may also become low.
Wanting to escape	The fight-or-flight response is well tuned: if we can't fight, now it's time to flee.	Self-preservation – we are programmed to survive.
Calming down, fleeing, fainting	Fainting may be protective; it feigns death. The body is taking care of itself, doing what it is programmed to do.	After fainting or escaping, breathing and heart rates slow, and blood flow and oxygen levels to the brain return to normal.

Why do I panic if there is no danger?

When we examine the number of body systems involved, it is not surprising that panic attacks are so debilitating, nor that they are dreaded by people who experience them. Even the thought of having another panic attack is frightening for people who have experienced one already, and they will do almost anything to avoid further attacks. Just thinking about a threat or danger in situations when there is no actual danger may activate the fight-or-flight response – even in people who do not experience panic attacks. For example, watching a scary movie or thinking about a frightening, stressful or dangerous situation that happened in the past may be enough to trigger a cascade of hormones and activate the fight-or-flight response. We've all experienced a situation during a scary part of a film or TV program when our hearts start to pound and we can't bear to watch the screen, just as the villain is about to strike or the raft is about to go over the waterfall. Unfortunately for a person who is already over-breathing through stress or habit, just thinking about the latest panic attack may be enough to increase anxiety and stress levels. In addition, the survival instinct may be set on high alert, making some people more prone to panic.

If you examine Table 3.1 you can see that the body is reacting in a protective way during a panic attack and is doing what we are all primed to do when the fight-or-flight response is activated. Although the breathing pattern may be disordered and the over-breathing is triggering the panic symptoms, the body is doing its best to help us to avoid harm.

FAMOUS PEOPLE AND PANIC

If you experience anxiety and panic, you are not alone. Many famous people, including artists, writers and celebrities, have suffered from these conditions. Charles Darwin, the well-known nineteenth-century English naturalist and geologist, was often ill during his life, mainly in times of stress and over-work. He acknowledged that his health always deteriorated from the excitement of going into society, particularly on occasions such as attending meetings or making social visits. His symptoms appear to be those related to anxiety and panic, and included stomach problems, vomiting, nervous dyspepsia, headaches, palpitations and trembling, shivering and faintness. In recent times there have been several theories as to what Darwin actually suffered from, and a number of sources point to panic disorder and agoraphobia (fear of open spaces).[12] From the symptoms listed, it's possible that Darwin did suffer from anxiety and panic, although we'll never know for sure.

Darwin studied evolution and is well known for his work on natural selection. One famous quote attributed to him (but not actually said by Darwin) is: 'It is not the strongest of the species that survives, nor the most intelligent, but the ones most responsive to change.'[13] Are the anxiety and panic symptoms that some people experience part of our evolutionary adaptation and therefore necessary for our survival as a species? We could contend that we need to have that extra level of alertness built in (for some people) to ensure survival of the species. Although we all have a survival instinct, theoretically, in times of danger, one or two *hypervigilant* people could ensure the safety of the entire tribe. It's a question Darwin would probably have loved to ponder if only he had known about anxiety and adrenaline: Darwin died in 1882 and the fight-or-flight hormone, adrenaline, was not identified until 1902.[14]

Adrenaline and its role in over-breathing, anxiety and panic is now well established and documented in medical literature. Although there are exceptions,[15] retraining the breathing pattern as a modality to reduce or eliminate these conditions is not generally well known or given the prominence it deserves.

CHAPTER 4

Hyperventilation syndrome

A forgotten, invisible illness

Lisa was in her teens when her mother enrolled her in a breathing retraining course. She had been diagnosed with hyperventilation syndrome and panic disorder a few months prior to her enrolment. A course of anti-anxiety medication and counselling had not been effective. The list of symptoms Lisa experienced was frightening, especially for one so young: anxiety, panic attacks, migraines, shortness of breath, difficulty in breathing, dizziness, insomnia, tingling in extremities and stress, to name just a few. Over-breathing dominated and controlled every aspect of Lisa's young life: studies, sports, hobbies, daily activities and even sleep.

No mother wants to see her child suffer in this way. Lisa's mother was very resourceful and googled some key words such as 'hyperventilation', which led her to my practice.

When I met Lisa, she appeared very despondent and defeated. She was slumped forwards and she looked pale and tired with dark circles under her eyes. She was not obviously over-breathing, although I noticed that when she spoke she seemed to take deeper breaths, and from time to time she yawned. When we looked at Lisa's breathing assessment using a capnometer, Lisa's carbon dioxide levels indicated severe over-breathing – one of the most severe cases I had seen in years of practice. No wonder Lisa had so many symptoms.

After following the breathing retraining guidelines overnight, Lisa reported that she had slept well and felt more clear-headed. By day four of the course Lisa was beginning to improve further. And when Lisa and her mother returned for a follow-up review a couple of weeks after the course, Lisa looked very different: smiling, vivacious and healthy, and her posture was great! The dark circles under her eyes were gone, and so was that tired, grey pallor.

It was not surprising, therefore, that a breathing assessment now showed that Lisa's end-tidal carbon dioxide levels were almost in the normal range. I asked Lisa to take a red pen and mark an X beside any of the symptoms she no longer experienced. Lisa thoughtfully placed red Xs beside most of the symptoms she had ticked prior to her course, including panic attacks, insomnia, stress, shortness of breath and migraines.

How could I not love my work?

What is hyperventilation syndrome?

Hyperventilation syndrome (HVS) is a chronic breathing-related condition that is very rarely mentioned and, I suspect, is vastly under-diagnosed. In fact, we could call it 'the forgotten, invisible illness'. Severe and prolonged over-breathing in HVS causes imbalances in body chemistry, which lead to numerous physical and psychological symptoms, as shown in Table 4.1 (on page 47). HVS may be psychologically or physiologically based – in other words, there may be an underlying stress or anxiety – or it may be due to over-breathing, which starts during a stressful period or event and subsequently becomes a habit.

According to a review by the prestigious Cochrane Collaboration, it's estimated that a staggering 9.5 per cent of the general adult population suffers from dysfunctional breathing/HVS.[1, 2] The incidence of this condition is almost on a par with that of asthma, which is 10.8 per cent according to the Australian Bureau of Statistics,[3] yet most people have never even heard of dysfunctional breathing or HVS. The sad part is that many people may unknowingly be suffering from HVS – a condition where breathing retraining is effective in improving health and eliminating the numerous symptoms that are inevitably present.

According to stress and anxiety expert Professor Robert Fried, hyperventilation or over-breathing is probably the most common of the stress-related breathing disorders.[4] Various estimates suggest that over-breathing is considered to occur in approximately 10–25 per cent of the general population, although not all of these people will develop the severe over-breathing that is part of hyperventilation syndrome. However, it would not be surprising if hyperventilation syndrome is vastly under-diagnosed, given these high estimates for over-breathing in the general population.

In HVS, over-breathing contributes to a large number of physical and psychological symptoms and conditions that may seem apparently unrelated to breathing – or to each other. For example, over-breathing may cause constriction in arterial blood vessels, which may restrict blood to the heart, causing angina and chest pain. Further, an association between hyperventilation and conditions such as migraines and idiopathic (i.e. with no known cause) seizures has been described.[5] Yet we very rarely – if ever – hear about the association between over-breathing and these disorders.

My young client Lisa had been diagnosed with hyperventilation syndrome and had experienced numerous symptoms, including panic attacks. Lisa may have been fortunate to receive a diagnosis, but it wasn't until her breathing retraining course that she saw an improvement in her symptoms.

A plethora of unrelated symptoms

People who suffer from HVS usually have a long list of seemingly unrelated signs and symptoms, as depicted in Table 4.1. But make no mistake: these symptoms are all related to over-breathing. Fortunately, people with this condition do not experience all of the symptoms in this table, but those they do experience are usually severe and can affect quality of life. Often, despite extensive medical investigations and tests, people who are actually suffering from HVS discover to their surprise and consternation that everything appears normal and nothing is found to account for their various symptoms.

In its extreme form, hyperventilation can be associated with tetany, a condition that involves twitching, cramping and spasms in the extremities due to very low carbon dioxide levels, and alkalosis, a condition that occurs when the system becomes too alkaline due to extremely low carbon dioxide levels.

Surprisingly, as in Lisa's story, obvious over-breathing may not be apparent in many people suffering from HVS. Some people with this condition may have a pattern of taking occasional deep breaths, combined with sighing or yawning, which tends to mask any obvious signs of over-breathing such as loud, noisy breathing. Decreased carbon dioxide levels may be present without any obvious change in air intake or breathing volume, if the person sighs or yawns frequently and the sighs and yawns are interspersed with normal respirations.[6] It is not necessary to mouth-breathe or even to take loud, noisy or bigger breaths in order to over-breathe and reduce carbon dioxide levels sufficiently to cause symptoms.

Although HVS may be common, it is often overlooked as a cause or a contributor to stress, anxiety and panic symptoms. Adding to the confusion is the fact that the over-breathing may be intermittent and is not always picked up on observation, or during testing, of the patient.[7] Given the long list of potential and apparently unrelated signs and symptoms shown in Table 4.1, it's no wonder that this condition even has some experts baffled.

We can see from this list why HVS may be so difficult to diagnose and why patients may do the rounds and see several specialists, and may even have extensive and/or invasive tests before they get a diagnosis. If they are fortunate enough to receive a diagnosis, that is – I suspect that many patients may never receive a diagnosis (except perhaps 'anxiety') for their condition.

With HVS, erratic breathing patterns such as breath holding, excessive sighing and yawning may be seen and the person may complain of 'air hunger', difficulty in breathing or shortness of breath, as in over-breathing generally. However, with HVS, over-breathing may also result in many severe and troublesome symptoms such as a feeling of breathlessness, chest tightness, headaches, dizziness, tremor, faintness, a feeling of apprehension and tingling in the extremities, to name just a few.[8]

Several of the symptoms on the list in Table 4.1 (on the next page) are directly related to breathing, but most are not obvious and may appear to be totally unrelated. For example, HVS symptoms may appear in the stomach, the heart, the brain and the nervous system. Therefore, the person may be referred to a respiratory specialist for difficulty in breathing, a gastroenterologist for bloating and distension, a heart specialist for palpitations and chest tightness or chest pain, a neurologist for headaches, dizziness and faintness, or a psychiatrist because they have so many troublesome symptoms and nothing is showing up in their investigations.

HVS is a condition with a very interesting history. It was first described during the American Civil War by the physician Dr Jacob Mendes Da Costa, where soldiers with mysterious symptoms were said to be suffering from 'irritable heart' or Da Costa's Syndrome. Later, during World War I, it was called 'soldier's heart' or 'shell-shock'. However, it was not until 1937 that doctors Kerr, Dalton and Gliebe coined the term 'hyperventilation syndrome'.[9]

From this history, we can see that ongoing or profound stress is a precipitating factor. In HVS, the over-breathing habit that started during a very stressful period, continues *after* the stress has ended and may become severe, giving rise to numerous symptoms.

TABLE 4.1: POTENTIAL HYPERVENTILATION SYNDROME SIGNS AND SYMPTOMS[10]	
General	Weakness, fatigue, exhaustion Irritability, emotional outbursts Frightening dreams Insomnia, sleep issues Unable to tolerate stressors Blurred vision Headaches, migraines
Lungs and breathing	Breathlessness, air hunger, shortness of breath Difficulty in breathing Cough Chronic throat tickle Asthma-like symptoms Breath holding Chest tightness, chest pain Excessive sighing Excessive yawning
Muscles and skeleton	Muscle aches Muscle spasm Stiffness Joint pain Tremors/twitching/shivering Spasm of feet or hands
The nervous system	Dizziness, faintness, blackout Loss of balance Confusion, disorientation Impaired concentration, impaired judgement Impaired memory Poor analytical capacity Sense of unreality, feeling 'spaced' Feeling of losing one's mind Tingling, numbness and coldness of fingers, face and feet Sweaty palms, cold hands Seizures
The heart and blood vessels	Palpitations Skipped heartbeats Rapid pulse Aching in lower ribs

TABLE 4.1: POTENTIAL HYPERVENTILATION SYNDROME SIGNS AND SYMPTOMS[10]	
The digestive system	Dry mouth
	A feeling of swelling or a lump in the throat
	Difficulty in swallowing
	Abdominal cramps
	Bloating, swallowing air, belching
	Flatulence
	Distension
	Nausea
	Soreness in upper abdomen or stomach area
Mental and psychological	Anxiety
	Tension
	Apprehension
	Panic

There is a difference between hyperventilation, which means over-breathing (either intermittently or chronically), and HVS, where the hyperventilation is severe and sustained and may affect several of the body's organs and systems.

> At one end of the over-breathing spectrum are stress and anxiety, while at the extreme end is multiple organ involvement with numerous – apparently unrelated – symptoms and no abnormality found on medical tests.

Although the estimated incidence of HVS is around 10 per cent, there are concerns that the number of diagnosed cases may represent just the tip of the clinical iceberg, with many patients' symptoms going unrecognised and, therefore, untreated.[11]

People experiencing HVS seem to fall into the cracks between medicine and psychiatry. As Professor Robert Fried comments, 'Medicine generally recognises the symptoms of hyperventilation syndrome but it attributes them to anxiety, while psychiatry holds the very same set of symptoms to indicate subconscious conflict translated into psychophysiological [mind-body] disorders.'[12]

It's worth looking at some of the symptoms in more detail. A dry mouth, belching, bloating, flatulence, distension and epigastric or stomach pain are considered to occur in HVS due to swallowing of air while mouth-breathing. There is even a medical word used to describe swallowing air: 'aerophagy'.[13]

Headaches and over-breathing

Headaches are common in people who over-breathe and also in HVS. These range from a tiredness headache due to lack of sleep, through to tension headaches, blocked noses and sinus headaches, and probably the worst headaches: migraines. Even without all the other symptoms associated with HVS, migraine headaches alone would be enough to make life extremely difficult.

Frequent and severe headaches can take all the joy out of life and significantly reduce quality of life.

Tension, stress and posture

We all feel stressed occasionally and we may develop a tension headache from increased concentration or challenging events, for example, an exam or an interview, or from pressure at work. Tightness and tension in the neck and shoulder muscles arises after prolonged stress or from anxiety, and may also occur when sitting for prolonged periods in front of a computer screen.

When the pressures of work or study are extensive or excessive, and the stress levels and anxiety levels are significantly increased, this type of headache may develop more frequently. Improving the breathing pattern and reducing stress and tension are key to reducing this type of headache.

However, one cause of headaches that is not usually considered or mentioned is poor posture, and Lisa's posture was very poor. A slumping posture with the head thrust forwards, or with the shoulders raised and tense, may contribute to headaches. Tension in the head, jaw, neck or shoulders may contribute to headaches and exacerbate symptoms.

Having your vision checked is also recommended if you are having frequent headaches. Headaches can also be related to dehydration, so it's worthwhile keeping an eye on your water consumption.

Let's take a look at the different types of headaches and how they may relate to breathing.

Sinus headaches

This type of headache is mostly associated with mouth-breathing and a blocked nose. There may be dark circles under the eyes. Occasionally there may be an infection in the sinuses. Following a night of mouth-breathing, the person may wake up with a dry mouth, a blocked nose and a frontal headache, which extends from the forehead to below the eyes and into the cheeks, i.e. the area of the sinuses. There may be mucus or secretions blocking the nasal passages and the sinuses. I have found from my practice that when the breathing pattern improves and the person is nose-breathing comfortably, particularly at night, this type of headache can be eliminated.

Migraine headaches

Migraine headaches are excruciating and can prevent us from performing our everyday activities for hours or even days, having a serious impact on our quality of life. Migraine headaches are generally severe, throbbing headaches, sometimes on one side of the head. They may start with visual disturbances, described as an aura, such as bright lights, specks or flashes, or lines or shapes that come into the visual field. Migraines can last a few hours, or even for up to seventy-two hours in severe cases. There may be nausea and vomiting during the attacks, and afterwards the person feels washed out and drained.[14]

The cause of migraine headaches is unknown, but they are thought to be related to alteration or disturbances in the arterial blood vessels in the head or abdomen. They may also be linked to over-breathing. Spasms in blood vessels to the brain may be related to the reduced carbon dioxide levels associated with over-breathing. Therefore, it may be argued that there is a high probability of headache in people who are over-breathing, and I have found from my practice that migraines are common in people experiencing stress, anxiety and panic symptoms.

In fact, studies have shown that panic disorder is more strongly associated with migraines than most other anxiety disorders. The odds of having panic disorder are almost four times greater among people with migraines than those without.[15]

Recent research has also shown that there is an increased risk of migraines in people with asthma.[16] Asthma is another condition that involves over-breathing.

The severity of migraines may be reduced if the person manages to get to them early enough and takes an anti-nausea medication and a pain relief medication to help ward off the attack. There are also specific anti-migraine medications available via prescription from a doctor. Take care: frequent use of some over-the-counter pain relief medications for headaches may have side effects such as stomach inflammation or ulcers.

Some foods may be implicated in migraine headaches and some people may have food intolerances to items such as dairy, wheat, red wine or additives. If you suffer from migraines, it may be worthwhile keeping a diary of food and drink consumed to see if there is a pattern. Others may develop a migraine if they have been fasting for a few hours, and there appears to be an association between low blood sugar (hypoglycaemia) and migraines.

Despite efforts to raise awareness of migraines in the community, it is estimated that around 50 per cent of people with severe or frequent migraines do not receive professional treatment.[17]

The bottom line is if you are experiencing frequent headaches or migraines, it is worthwhile assessing your breathing pattern using the questionnaire in the next chapter. Also, please consult your doctor.

Fortunately, the majority of my clients manage to eliminate or reduce their headaches with breathing retraining. Improvements in breathing pattern and in sleep combined with a reduction in stress levels can make a significant difference in eliminating headaches.

Finding relief from HVS

Despite the statistics, in my experience HVS does seem to be fairly rare – or, to be more specific, rarely diagnosed – whereas anxiety and panic disorders are more commonly diagnosed conditions. However, there is a great deal of overlap between panic disorder and HVS. According to some estimates, 25 per cent of patients diagnosed with HVS also have symptoms of panic disorder.[18] Perhaps even more confusing, HVS, like over-breathing in general, may be intermittent or chronic.

Although generalised anxiety disorder, panic disorder and HVS share many similarities, from a medical and psychological perspective they are generally viewed as separate conditions. Although stress-related, the exact cause of HVS may be unknown but there appears to be a higher incidence among first-degree relatives than in the general population.[19]

According to a 2013 expert review by the Cochrane Collaboration, there is little consensus regarding the most effective management of HVS. In addition, this review states that no conclusions could be drawn to guide medical practice on breathing retraining because no credible evidence regarding the effectiveness of breathing exercises for HVS was found.[20] By 'credible' the authors mean well-designed, randomised, controlled trials with adequate numbers of participants that would meet the eligibility criteria of the review. As far as I am aware, none of the trials considered by the review panel included trials of the Buteyko method for HVS, as these have not been conducted.[21] (To date, trials of the Buteyko method have focused on asthma.)

When we think of signs and symptoms, we need to think of body systems as being highly interrelated. What occurs in one system affects other systems, and this is especially pertinent for over-breathing. From practical experience, the optimum way to improve the breathing pattern in HVS is to do a breathing retraining course with an accredited and experienced breathing retraining practitioner. The techniques and guidelines in Part 2 of this book may also be extremely effective in reducing or eliminating symptoms. In addition, if there are unresolved psychological conflicts or issues, counselling may be appropriate.

> The sheer number of symptoms in relation to several different organs and body systems, combined with negative findings on medical tests, may be a red flag for hyperventilation syndrome.

A prominent and well-known online guide for healthcare professionals suggests the following measures to treat HVS: supportive counselling, sometimes psychiatric or psychological treatment, and reassurance. While reassurance that the condition is not life threatening may be helpful, most people experiencing so many symptoms need practical assistance, not just reassurance. Possibly because of the lack of clinical trials, there is no mention of breathing retraining for HVS in this online guide despite it being a condition where over-breathing is the underlying cause and the main contributor to symptoms. This guide also suggests that some healthcare professionals advocate teaching the patient 'maximal exhalation and diaphragmatic breathing'. I question the rationale behind this – if someone is already over-breathing and exhaling excessive amounts of carbon dioxide, then maximal exhalation may not be appropriate.

Breathing into a paper bag for a short time, once traditionally used as a remedy for panic attacks, is not recommended for HVS. The rationale was that the person rebreathed the exhaled carbon dioxide from the bag and this helped to calm the breathing down. Nowadays this practice is rarely used, as it is not considered safe, practical or appealing. At worst, it may be risky or hazardous. For example, this is not a safe practice if someone is over-breathing due to a medical condition or has a heart condition or asthma. Also, it's not something most people would want to do in public or when under pressure at work.

If you are experiencing numerous symptoms and you suspect that you may be suffering from HVS, I recommend that you consult a doctor. If you then have a confirmed diagnosis of HVS, a breathing retraining course with an experienced practitioner or, alternatively, following the recommendations in Part 2 may provide considerable relief from symptoms. If you have already gone down the path of specialist after specialist, and have been told that all tests are negative, then following these recommendations may be very effective in calming your breathing pattern down and alleviating symptoms. If you decide to consult a breathing retraining practitioner, care is needed in choosing a practitioner; please see Appendix 1 for details and recommendations.

Without appropriate treatment, HVS can continue for years and may result in very poor health and also poor quality of life. But the experience of my young client Lisa is fairly typical of most people with severe breathing issues who do a breathing retraining course. The majority of people will experience improvement in their breathing pattern and reduced symptoms during the first week of breathing retraining, but it will generally take a number of weeks to consolidate the improved breathing pattern.

CHAPTER 5

Assess your breathing

The Breathing Questionnaire

'After I spoke to you on the phone I sat down and had a good cry. Here at last was someone who understood, and who was going to help me. I realised you knew what you were talking about as soon as you mentioned "air hunger".' These were among Jo's first words to me at the beginning of her breathing retraining course.

Jo loves her work but she has a challenging career and was experiencing frequent anxiety and panic attacks, which, despite medical treatment, had been going on for a few months. When I asked Jo if there were situations when her symptoms were better or worse, she replied, 'I have some better days, but they're there all day, every day!'

When I assessed Jo's breathing using a capnometer, Jo said that she was having one of her rare 'better' days. However, capnometry showed that Jo's carbon dioxide levels were reduced and indicated that she was moderately over-breathing. This meant that she was inhaling an increased volume of air and as a result was also exhaling excessive amounts of carbon dioxide.

In addition, the capnograph showed that instead of a nice regular breathing pattern, Jo had an irregular breathing pattern.

On her breathing assessment questionnaire, Jo ticked several boxes, including tiredness, frequent sighing and yawning, and mouth-breathing, as well as sleep issues. She also ticked the boxes for shortness of breath and tightness in the chest.

Following her capnometry and breathing assessment questionnaire, Jo was surprised but also relieved to find that there was an identifiable cause for her anxiety and panic symptoms: over-breathing. She enrolled in the next available breathing retraining course.

At first, Jo found the breathing exercises quite hard work and her progress seemed slow. But she persevered and, within a couple of weeks, she had improved considerably. Her posture, which had been poor, improved. And as her sleep improved, Jo's energy and concentration levels also gradually improved.

When Jo returned for her follow-up review, her breathing pattern during capnometry assessment looked so regular she was amazed and delighted! I was also pleased to see that her carbon dioxide levels had improved and were in the normal to optimal range, which meant that she was no longer over-breathing. Best of all, she had experienced only one panic attack in four weeks. 'I learnt to recognise when my breathing was off, and then I took action to prevent the attacks from happening. I took a few minutes of quiet time or time out to practise the exercises and to calm down my breathing,' she told me. Not only had retraining calmed her breathing but she said it had also calmed down her racing thoughts, which had been all over the place and affecting her sleep.

Happy and feeling calm, Jo was well on the road to recovery.

If you experience anxiety or panic symptoms on a regular basis, like Jo in the scenario above, you may be aware that your breathing pattern is somehow disordered, and you may assume that your anxiety or panic symptoms are affecting your breathing pattern. But what if it's the other way round? What if your breathing pattern is actually causing, triggering or even perpetuating your symptoms? Has anyone suggested that you need to test your breathing pattern?

In fact, there is a screening test to detect hyperventilation that has been around for more than thirty years. It's called the Nijmegen Questionnaire. But this test was developed mainly for hyperventilation syndrome and there is some debate about whether it is appropriate for use in other conditions, such as asthma.[1]

I developed a fairly comprehensive breathing questionnaire many years ago, without seeing the Nijmegen Questionnaire or even being aware of its existence, I have to confess. The questionnaire that I use is more concerned with some of the practicalities of over-breathing, e.g. mouth-breathing, although it also focuses on the signs and symptoms of over-breathing, as in the Nijmegen Questionnaire.

It's interesting for me to see that Jo, like many of my clients, had suspected for years that her breathing was not quite right and she had assumed that her anxiety symptoms and her panic attacks were causing the chest tightness, shortness of breath and the feeling of air hunger she experienced on a daily basis. When Jo completed the breathing questionnaire, she was surprised to find that it was her disordered breathing pattern that was triggering her symptoms.

Table 5.1 (on page 62) contains the questionnaire I use with my clients to assess their breathing pattern before they start their breathing retraining course. I recommend that you take the time to complete the questionnaire to see what your breathing pattern is really like. All it takes is a couple of minutes. If you tick the 'Don't know' box for some of the questions – for example, if you are not sure if you snore, or if your breathing is audible, or if you mouth-breathe – then you could ask your partner or a close friend or family member what they think. You may be surprised at their responses. Feel free to complete the questionnaire now or when you are ready to start the breathing retraining recommendations set out in Part 2 of this book. You can make two copies of this questionnaire, so that you can monitor your progress later.

It may sometimes be difficult for people to assess what their breathing is really like. Generally, we are not aware of our breathing and we don't always notice what is happening, as breathing is so instinctive. Sometimes at the start of the breathing retraining course, clients will tell me, 'I always breathe through my nose!' when I can see quite clearly that this is not accurate. At an opportune moment I have to gently point out that they are mouth-breathing, which sometimes comes as a huge surprise. They may also have an audible, sighing type of respiration and may not realise that this is part of a disordered breathing pattern.

In addition, they may be gulping air as they speak and/or taking huge breaths at the end of their sentences, which they are also not aware of. Their breathing may be noisy and can be heard from across the room, yet they may not be aware of this either. Female partners (it's usually women!) will say, 'I can hear him breathing from the next room.' And because the person has breathed this way for so long, they may think there is nothing wrong with their breathing pattern.

Guidelines for the breathing questionnaire

The questions in the breathing questionnaire need to be interpreted as what occurs on a regular basis with your 'normal' breathing pattern – not when you are exercising, or if you have a cold or flu, when it would be more likely for you to feel short of breath or for your nose to block or to have an increase in mucus.

Please tick the boxes as follows:

Rarely may be interpreted as hardly ever occurring; perhaps up to three times a year.

Occasionally means now and then, perhaps once a month.

Frequently means several times a week or daily.

Please note: this questionnaire is for information only and is not intended for diagnosis of any condition. Please consult your doctor for a clinical assessment and diagnosis.

TABLE 5.1: ASSESS YOUR BREATHING QUESTIONNAIRE

Make two copies of this questionnaire –
one for the start and one for the end of your program.

Tick your answers to the following questions (see guidelines in the text)

Never = N | Rarely = R | Occasionally = O | Frequently = F | Don't know = DK

		N	R	O	F	DK
1.	Does your breathing feel uncomfortable?					
2.	Can you hear yourself breathe?					
3.	Do you breathe through your mouth?					
4.	Do you feel your upper chest move when taking a breath?					
5.	Does your nose block?					
6.	Do you get post-nasal drip?					
7.	Do you find it difficult to nose-breathe?					
8.	Do you sneeze excessively?					
9.	Do you wheeze?					
10.	Do you take deep breaths through the mouth when speaking?					
11.	Do you cough excessively or get a tickly cough?					
12.	Do you need to blow your nose excessively?					
13.	Do you experience a lack of energy?					
14.	Do you feel stressed?					
15.	Do you experience anxiety?					
16.	Do you sigh or yawn excessively?					
17.	Do you get shortness of breath or chest tightness?					
18.	Do you snore?					
19.	Do you wake up with a dry mouth or need to keep water by your bedside?					
20.	Do you experience headaches or wake up with a headache?					
21.	Do you experience a lack of concentration?					
22.	Do you experience irritability?					
23.	Do you experience tiredness?					
24.	Do you experience dizziness or feel spaced?					
25.	Do you lose your sense of smell?					
26.	Do you get tingling in your fingers?					
27.	Do you get palpitations?					

Check your results

Please bear in mind that no test is ever 100 per cent accurate. However, I find the breathing questionnaire provides a very good indication of my clients' breathing patterns. To obtain a diagnosis, however, you will need to consult a doctor. Of course, if you haven't seen your doctor for a check-up, you will need to do this before assuming that your symptoms are entirely breathing related, as a number of medical conditions can contribute to increased breathing.

- **All ticks in the Never column:**
  Congratulations! It sounds like your breathing pattern is fine.

- **Mostly ticked the Never and Rarely columns:**
  Your breathing pattern may need to be improved. For example, if you ticked that you wheeze or get palpitations or tingling in your fingers – even on rare occasions – this is not part of a normal breathing pattern.

- **Mostly ticked the Rarely or Occasionally columns:**
  Your breathing pattern may be affecting your health and could do with some improvement. Any ticks in the Occasionally column may point to a disordered breathing pattern, particularly if you say that your breathing is uncomfortable or if you mouth-breathe. The more ticks you have in the Occasionally column, the more likely it is that you may be over-breathing, either chronically or intermittently.

- **Mostly ticked the Occasionally column but some in the Frequently column:**
  Your breathing pattern is probably affecting your health and needs to be improved. The more ticks you have in the Frequently column, the more likely it is that you may be over-breathing either intermittently or chronically.

- **Several ticks in the Frequently column:**
  Your breathing pattern may be seriously affecting your health and your quality of life. You may be chronically over-breathing, and improving your breathing pattern will improve your health. If you ticked Frequently in response to question 19 (*Do you wake up with a dry mouth or need to keep water by your bedside?*), this generally indicates that you are mouth-breathing – and over-breathing – and, therefore, most likely over-breathing during the daytime as well.

- **Mostly ticked the Frequently column:**
  You may suspect or even be aware that your breathing pattern may be significantly disordered. So the fact that you could be over-breathing may not come as a total surprise. Your breathing pattern is probably affecting your health, mood, sleep and quality of life. It may be affecting many aspects of your life and is possibly related to numerous symptoms. You need to take steps to improve your breathing pattern.

Don't be alarmed or despondent if you have placed several ticks in the Frequently column of the breathing questionnaire. Most of my clients with anxiety and panic symptoms tick several of the Frequently boxes at the start of their breathing retraining course. In fact, in my practice, the number of ticks clients place in the Frequently column is almost a predictor of reduced end-tidal carbon dioxide levels when we do the capnometry assessment. And as you will learn from reading this book, you can be optimistic about changing your breathing pattern and improving your symptoms. While this questionnaire may be somewhat subjective and open to interpretation, in practice I find that it provides a very good indication of clients' breathing patterns.

Questions relating to sleep, tiredness and lack of energy

If you ticked Frequently for questions 13, 18, 19, 20, 21, 22, and/or 23, your breathing pattern is probably affecting your sleep, leaving you fatigued, irritable and unable to concentrate during the day, and this lack of quality sleep may be contributing to your daytime symptoms and to increased stress. If you ticked Frequently to questions 13 (lack of energy) and 23 (tiredness), this may also be related to over-breathing and to poor sleep quality. However, there are hundreds of other reasons for chronic tiredness, so this should be checked by your doctor.

It can be a bit confronting to learn that your breathing pattern needs to be improved. At this stage, it's not unusual to feel deflated or even a little angry – at yourself for not realising what was happening, or at your healthcare providers who perhaps did not identify the breathing issues. It may not sound like good news, but the fact is if you have identified that your breathing pattern is disordered and needs attention, then you've taken a step in the right direction. My clients are sometimes surprised or even shocked initially to discover that they are over-breathing, but they are also relieved to find that there is something physical – or physiological, to be more precise – i.e. over-breathing, contributing to their symptoms and that it can be improved or even eliminated.

It really doesn't matter how, when or why the anxiety or panic symptoms (or the over-breathing) started. Dwelling on the past is not productive, unless you are receiving professional counselling. The objective now is to learn how to improve your breathing pattern so that you don't continue to overreact to stress and perpetuate the cycle.

Monitor your progress

You will want to see how much progress you are making during the four weeks of the breathing retraining program in Part 2 of this book. The breathing questionnaire can be repeated at the end of your program to check your progress. I find that people quickly forget that they had some symptoms and are sometimes surprised when I show them what they ticked initially!

CHAPTER 6

The myth of deep breathing

'I thought deep breathing was good for us!'

Fay is a fit, active and apparently healthy woman in her late twenties who attended my practice. But Fay's enrolment form told a very different story: this young woman had a multitude of symptoms – including anxiety, panic attacks, waking at night and migraines – which she had been experiencing for more than six months and which she had attributed to stress. Fay had been diagnosed with panic disorder by her doctor.

Fay was also constantly mouth-breathing. Her nose kept blocking and she was continually struggling for air. Naturally, Fay was very concerned; she couldn't figure out why she was experiencing so many symptoms.

As usual, I assessed Fay's breathing using a capnometer. Fay's end-tidal carbon dioxide levels were found to be low and indicated moderately severe over-breathing. In addition, Fay's respiration rate at rest was 20 per minute, which is rather fast (optimal is 8–14 per minute for an adult). Fay's resting pulse rate was also quite high for an apparently fit and healthy young woman, at 85–90 beats per minute.

Fay's posture was also poor: she was slumped forwards. I could see that she was breathing from the top of her chest and she was not using her diaphragm correctly.

Fay was rather sceptical when I explained that she was over-breathing. 'I thought deep breathing was good for us!' she said in amazement.

When I explained that over-breathing was causing and contributing to her symptoms, Fay was eager to get started on the breathing retraining exercises. She was aware that she was mouth-breathing and she found nose-breathing quite difficult initially. Improving posture to allow effective use of the diaphragm was also high on the list of objectives and Fay gradually became more aware of her posture. By the end of the week, Fay's symptoms were improving and she found that her breathing was becoming easier.

One month later, Fay attended for a follow-up review. She reported that she was sleeping much better and, in fact, she looked more relaxed. Fay's breathing assessment this time was very different: her breathing rate had reduced to 13 breaths per minute and her end-tidal carbon dioxide levels were now not just normal but in the optimal range. Her heart rate was a healthy 72 beats per minute.

Best of all, Fay was no longer experiencing anxiety and panic attacks, and the migraines were a thing of the past.

How could deep breathing be so bad?

Most of us assume that deep breathing is good for us – it's what we were all brought up to believe. From kindergarten to senior citizens' groups, at school or at a conference, we are all familiar with the standard advice: 'Stand up and take nice big breaths!' Or: 'Take a deep breath in and blow it all off ... see how good that feels?' This belief in the power of deep breathing has been the prevailing – and mainly unchallenged – conventional wisdom for most of our lives.

Yet the truth is very different. There is absolutely no evidence to support the contention that deep breathing is good for us; in fact, for some people who are already over-breathing, it can be very bad indeed, and may exacerbate symptoms such as stress, anxiety and panic.

The claim that deep breathing is good for us is one of the greatest myths perpetrated throughout most of the twentieth century and into the twenty-first century.

If you are like the majority of people and have always believed that deep breathing is good for you, prepare to have this belief seriously challenged.

Claims that deep breathing is good for us and that we need to breathe deeply in order to get more oxygen in are two of the greatest myths perpetrated throughout most of the twentieth century and into the twenty-first century. In fact, the reverse is true – the deeper we breathe, the less oxygen reaches the cells and tissues. This belief in the benefits of deep breathing is possibly due to a westernised version of eastern practices such as yoga and meditation, which were popularised in the latter half of the twentieth century and whose traditions then made their way into conventional wisdom, largely accepted unquestioned by the general population, and even by healthcare professionals such as myself.

This belief in the merits of deep breathing is something that I, as a registered nurse, accepted and adopted as a principle of professional practice. It was not until I read an article in *The Medical Journal of Australia* (*MJA*) in 1998[1] about the first trial of breathing retraining for asthma in the western world using the Buteyko method (developed by a Russian doctor, Konstantin Buteyko, in the 1950s) that I started to research and question the potential benefits or harms of deep breathing.

My research found absolutely nothing to support the idea that deep breathing is good for the average person, and to my consternation I found that deep breathing is not only *not* good for us, it may in fact may be *bad* for some people, particularly for those with conditions such as asthma, angina, anxiety and panic disorder. (I am not speaking here about patients in hospital or even at home who are on some medications such as strong pain relief that may reduce breathing, or who have recently had surgery or anaesthetics and whose breathing may be shallow, in which case the emphasis on breathing more deeply is, of course, appropriate and correct. I am referring instead to the average person in the community who may have had symptoms of stress, anxiety and panic for months or even decades.)

In a world where we are constantly taught that deep breathing is good for us, it is interesting to look more closely at anxiety and panic symptoms. Both may include shortness of breath, but does this mean that people with these conditions are not breathing deeply enough? On the contrary, the scientific evidence overwhelmingly shows that they are *over*-breathing, despite the fact that they may feel short of breath.

My client Fay was breathing rapidly and constantly trying to inhale more air, without success. She was also breathing through her mouth, which is generally not considered unusual in our society. But mouth-breathing is not a healthy way to breathe – the volume of air is increased when we mouth-breathe, and this increase in air volume leads to a disturbance in the balance of gases in the body and to adverse symptoms. Like many people, Fay did not relate her symptoms directly to her breathing pattern but attributed everything to stress. What she did not realise was that she was over-breathing considerably and this was causing symptoms and adding to her stress levels. When Fay normalised her breathing pattern through breathing retraining, the symptoms disappeared, as did the high stress levels.

Breathing pattern is a term that describes the way we breathe, and encompasses several different things, for example:

- The rate of breathing (the number of breaths per minute).
- Whether the breathing is regular or irregular.
- The depth of breathing (deep or shallow).
- Whether we are breathing gently or heavily.
- Whether we are mouth-breathing or nose-breathing.
- Whether the breathing is quiet or is noisy and audible.
- Whether we are adopting good posture or not.
- Whether we are breathing from the diaphragm or the chest.

- Whether the breathing is comfortable or not.
- Whether there is difficulty in breathing, such as shortness of breath.

As we saw in Table 1.1 in Chapter 1, normal breathing should be effortless, regular, and inaudible at rest (i.e. when seated or lying down), whereas when there is a disordered breathing pattern, the reverse is true. Struggling for air, difficulty in breathing, mouth-breathing, poor posture or audible breathing at rest are all regarded as part of a disordered breathing pattern (sometimes referred to as a dysfunctional breathing pattern). The pulse rate as well as the respiration rate may be increased. The normal adult pulse range is 50–80 beats per minute at rest, depending on fitness levels and how effective the heart is as a pump.

Breathing sustains us from birth, without us even having to think about it. Yet it is precisely because breathing is so instinctual that we are often not in tune with our breathing pattern; we accept disordered breathing because we have always breathed that way or possibly because our breathing pattern may have changed slowly over time without our being aware of the changes occurring.

The number one over-breathing habit

Do you breathe through your nose or your mouth?

Mouth-breathing is common in conditions such as stress, anxiety, panic, allergy, asthma, snoring, sleep-disordered breathing and a host of others. When we mouth-breathe, the volume of air inhaled is greatly increased. Constant mouth-breathing increases the volume of air by three or four times the normal level because the mouth allows a much greater volume of air to be inhaled than the nostrils – think of the difference between a drinking straw and a garden hose.

In fact, the volume of air we breathe can be measured in a lung function laboratory, but in my experience this is rarely done outside of clinical trials. This breathing test is called the 'minute volume' in medical terminology, and the adult range for resting minute volume (as seen in Table 6.1 overleaf) is 4–6 litres of air per minute. Minute volumes above this range while at rest, i.e. sitting or lying down, may indicate over-breathing. And, of course, it's not a case of one size fits all: a petite person will probably need to breathe a lesser volume of air than a tall, hefty person. It's all to do with the size of the person and the size of their lungs and their energy needs. Another factor is tidal volume. Tidal volume refers to the total volume of air inhaled with each breath – on average, around 500 ml per breath for adults. For example, 500 ml (tidal volume) multiplied by 12 breaths per minute provides a minute volume of 6000 ml or 6 litres as indicated in Table 6.1.[2] End-tidal carbon dioxide levels (discussed throughout this book) are a more objective way of assessing whether over-breathing is present.

We can also learn a lot just by observing a person's breathing and posture while they are unaware they are being observed. People tend to change their posture or even change the number of breaths per minute if they become aware of someone observing their breathing pattern (a bit like white-coat syndrome, where some patients' blood pressure shoots up as soon as the doctor or nurse tries to assess it!). When I trained as a nurse, I was taught that the best way to count the respiration rate is to pretend to be taking the pulse, while surreptitiously counting the number of breaths per minute. Optimal breathing and heart rates for an adult are provided in Table 6.1. However, counting your breaths per minute may not be accurate if you try to count them yourself, particularly if you are stressed or anxious.

TABLE 6.1: OPTIMAL RANGES (ADULTS)	
Heart rate	50–80 beats per minute
Breathing rate	8–14 breaths per minute
Minute volume	4–6 litres per minute
Tidal volume	500 ml per breath
End-tidal carbon dioxide levels	40–45 mmHg

When a person over-breathes, they can breathe in three or four times the normal volume of air but they may not even realise it. They may become aware of symptoms, some of which may seem unrelated to over-breathing, such as headaches, muscle tension, fatigue or even a blocked nose – and, of course, anxiety or panic. It is also possible to over-breathe while nose-breathing by increasing the number of breaths per minute or by taking deeper breaths or even by sighing or yawning excessively.

Of course, breathing is a dynamic process, and changes in the breathing pattern and the heart rate occur throughout the day and night, according to the activity or the situation. For example, after we eat our breathing rate and heart rate increase as we create the energy needed to digest our food. When we exercise, it's more obvious that the breathing rate is increased. If we are fighting off a virus and our body temperature is increased, breathing is also likely to be increased. In addition, when we are stressed or frightened, it is natural for breathing to increase. To use an extreme example, when running from a mad dog we would certainly feel the need to breathe more deeply or even to mouth-breathe, and the minute volume in that case would be considerably raised. This is a natural, albeit temporary, response to a fearful situation.

However, mouth-breathing is not necessarily a prerequisite for over-breathing. Some people experiencing anxiety and panic attacks rarely mouth-breathe. In this case there may be subtle clues. For example, the person may take more audible breaths while speaking, or their chest movements may be evident or their shoulders raised, as they breathe. These variations in breathing pattern were brought home to me many years ago when one of my clients attended a course of breathing retraining. Before the course, this gentleman was nose-breathing very loudly and could be heard from three metres away. Following the course, I could not hear his breathing as he sat right beside me.

For now, let me assure you that there is no research to support the claim that deep breathing is good for us. The notion of deep breathing as beneficial is a modern myth that has no foundation in research. For people who are already over-breathing, but may be unaware that they are over-breathing, deliberately deep breathing will increase symptoms and may lead to a worsening of their condition.

CHAPTER 7

Hidden hyperventilation

Anxiety states and fat-folder syndrome

Sarah phoned and said, 'I need help with my breathing – I keep holding my breath.' Although she appeared outwardly confident and well presented, I later discovered that Sarah was becoming extremely despondent and feeling more and more helpless. Sarah said that she was experiencing her 'little problem' (as she called it) on a regular basis. She could not even bring herself to acknowledge that what she meant was that she was regularly having anxiety and panic attacks, sometimes on a daily basis. The 'little problem' was ruling Sarah's life, as she relied heavily on her confidence in order to be able to carry out her work in a challenging career. Unfortunately, she was losing her confidence and, as a result, her life and work were becoming very stressful and difficult.

Sarah confided that although she had consulted her doctor, she had not been able to discuss her issues with her family or friends, as she found the situation too embarrassing. Sarah's symptoms were becoming worse as she tried to cope alone, and she was becoming more and more isolated.

It was only after Sarah's initial breathing assessment using capnometry showed that her end-tidal carbon dioxide levels were considerably reduced – which indicated moderate over-breathing – that Sarah began to grasp that this was not a question of managing or controlling the situation herself. Sarah could see her breathing pattern and her reduced carbon dioxide levels on the screen. She realised that this was a physical condition – a breathing issue, or, to be more precise, an over-breathing habit – which was increasing her stress levels and contributing to her symptoms.

Following a few ups and downs during her breathing retraining course, Sarah steadily improved, and at a follow-up appointment three weeks later she looked like a different person: cheerful, happy and relaxed. It was as if a huge weight had been lifted from her shoulders.

Sarah's end-tidal carbon dioxide levels were now normal and she was coping well with work. In addition, I was pleased to hear that she had spoken to members of her family and to some of her close friends about her experience. She reported that she was a little surprised, but also delighted, to find that they had been very understanding and sympathetic. 'After all,' Sarah said with a smile, 'why shouldn't I talk about it? It was just a breathing problem!'

Going it alone

Sarah's story is not uncommon. In fact, many of my clients are so embarrassed about their anxiety and panic attacks that they don't even speak about it to their family, friends or colleagues. They may eventually visit their doctor or see a psychologist, where they will have the opportunity to speak about their issues, but there is often a sense of shame or of personal failure. They may even be in denial, as Sarah was, in relation to their stress, anxiety and panic symptoms, so they try to tough it out alone. Not being able to talk about their issues adds to a person's stress levels and to their sense of isolation, and may even increase their symptoms and make their condition worse, as had occurred with Sarah.

The extent of this 'toughing it out' or 'going it alone' was brought home to me in one of my breathing retraining classes a few years ago. All of the three clients who had enrolled were experiencing stress, anxiety and panic attacks.

As a healthcare professional I am bound by professional ethics and I cannot refer to anyone's condition. So during classes, when I describe strategies to relieve a particular symptom, such as panic, I say, 'For those of you who have panic symptoms, I recommend the following,' and then describe the strategy. It was not until day four in a five-day course that one of my clients felt comfortable enough to acknowledge that she was experiencing panic attacks, which of course opened the floodgates, and the others admitted that they too were dealing with the same things.

To be able to talk openly about their issues in a small group was very helpful, and I could see my clients visibly relax and realise that what they had experienced was not unusual or a sign of weakness, as they may have thought. This experience really highlighted for me how isolating stress, anxiety and panic symptoms can be, and how unfair this is. If these people had been experiencing asthma symptoms or sleep apnoea, they would probably have talked openly about it on the first day of the course.

To disclose or not to disclose?

I am not advocating that if you are like my client Sarah and experience stress, anxiety and panic symptoms you should disclose your condition to everyone. In general, people are not well informed on this topic. You may need to be careful who you tell, as disclosure may put you under closer scrutiny in a work or study situation, for example. Disclosure in some circumstances can lead to increasing stress levels, which can in turn lead to a worsening of your symptoms.

However, mentioning the problem to a trusted family member or close friend may be helpful. Most people are sympathetic and understanding, as was the case with Sarah. Sharing the experience takes the pressure off and allows you to relax a little and not feel quite so isolated. It all depends on your circumstances. At the very least, you should be able to talk to a loved one or to your doctor or counsellor.

Hidden hyperventilation

In 1946, a young man named Konstantin Pavlovich Buteyko, from a farming family in Ivanitsa, a village near the city of Kiev in the Ukraine, enrolled to study medicine at the First Moscow Institute of Medicine. During his medical studies, an incident occurred that was to change the young man's life.

In the third year of his medical studies, Konstantin Buteyko was required to do an assignment on breathing as part of his studies. While working on this assignment, Buteyko asked a patient to breathe deeply to allow him to listen to and assess the patient's breathing. To Buteyko's surprise the patient fainted. Why had the patient fainted, when he was breathing deeply and apparently inhaling sufficient oxygen?[1]

Subsequently, Buteyko asked patients with asthma and angina to *reduce* their breathing in order for him to assess the effect. Angina is a type of chest pain related to insufficient blood flow to the heart muscle. Again to his surprise, the patients' symptoms were gone at once, Buteyko recalled. Then, when he asked the patients to breathe more deeply, their symptoms returned.

Buteyko realised he was on the verge of a major discovery. He asked himself why, in the history of medicine, had no-one thought of this previously. But Buteyko's teachers were not impressed when he shared his news. Illness cannot be improved by reducing breathing, they insisted. The discovery had piqued his interest, and Buteyko decided to research and develop techniques to retrain and improve breathing patterns.

Buteyko realised that without evidence his ideas would not be accepted. So he set about researching and proving his theory. From 1958 to 1959, he completed a study at the functional diagnostics research laboratory in the former Soviet Union's Meshalkin Institute, examining 200 people, both unwell and healthy. Buteyko's findings confirmed his theory on the correlation between hyperventilation and illness. In January 1960, Buteyko summed up his ideas in a report to members of a medical institute. Again, as in his student days, the response was stunned disbelief.[2]

Buteyko was ridiculed in his own country for his ideas.[3] It was not until three decades had passed and Konstantin Buteyko had run trials on thousands of patients that the Buteyko method was endorsed by the Soviet government as a mainstream approach to asthma management.[4]

Professor Buteyko discovered that over-breathing may not be obvious to the patient or to the doctor. Consequently, he called the condition 'hidden hyperventilation'. Further, he maintained that a great number of 'civilisation-induced diseases', as he called them, were caused by chronic over-breathing.[5] He contended that disorders due to over-breathing are aggravated by environmental pollution, pesticides and chemicals.

Professor Buteyko viewed over-breathing as a modern condition brought about by a number of causes, but mainly by misinformation on the benefits of deep breathing. His primary objective, he maintained, was to provide people with information on normal breathing in order to stop the focus on the advantages of deep breathing, which was (and still is) so prevalent in the mass media and in addition to withdraw deep-breathing exercises from healthcare institutions.[6]

Due to the Cold War, the Soviet Union was closed to the west, and it wasn't until 1990 that the work of Professor Buteyko became known outside of Russia, when it was brought to Sydney by one of Buteyko's protégés, Alexander Stalmatski. I was fortunate to be able to meet Professor Buteyko at a conference in New Zealand in 2000. He was then 78 years old. Despite the fact that he was probably jet-lagged after his flight from Moscow, he was extremely generous with his time and keen to spread the message and stop the dissemination of misinformation on the 'benefits' of deep breathing. Professor Buteyko was an advocate of getting back to basics and advised moderation in all things, such as eating less, sleeping less and normalising breathing – in other words, breathing less.

Professor Buteyko died in 2003, aged eighty. In a foreword to a 1997 book on the topic, he expressed the hope that, in time, a Buteyko practitioner would be found on every corner and that his treatment would be available to all.[7] These days there are practitioners throughout the world who follow his method, and several successful asthma trials on Buteyko's method have been conducted, but to date his hope for a practitioner 'on every corner' has not yet been realised.

However, some of Buteyko's ideas and recommendations are gradually coming to fruition. The deep-breathing philosophy is steadily losing ground in medicine and physiotherapy. Asthma patients are given advice to breathe gently, to nose-breathe and to avoid mouth-breathing on discharge from hospital after asthma attacks. This advice was not given fifteen or twenty years ago when deep breathing was still considered beneficial in this condition.

The tip of the iceberg

While Professor Buteyko conducted his research and developed his breathing retraining method behind the Iron Curtain, in England a respiratory physician and pioneer on hyperventilation research, the late Dr Claude Lum, was also studying the subject. Like Buteyko, Dr Lum asserted that hyperventilation was not always evident.

In a 1975 paper, Dr Lum referred to classic or obvious hyperventilation as 'the tip of the iceberg', occurring in only 1 per cent of cases.

> *The ninety-nine per cent who do not present in this fashion* [i.e. obviously hyperventilating] *(and are not accorded the dignity of a mention in any standard English text) presents a collection of bizarre and often apparently unrelated symptoms, which may affect any part of the body, and any organ or any system.*[8]

Dr Lum analysed the records of hundreds of hospital patients in England who had undergone numerous investigations because of their perplexing and troublesome symptoms without any abnormalities being found. These patients had somewhat callously been given the label 'anxiety states', based on the fact that no apparent organic cause for their symptoms could be identified. Some doctors dubbed these patients 'multiple doctor' patients, or as suffering from 'fat-folder syndrome' due to the thickness of their files and the number of investigations and procedures they had undergone.

However, when Dr Lum compared the symptoms of these so-called fat-folder syndrome patients with a group of patients who had been diagnosed with hyperventilation, he discovered that the symptoms of the two groups were virtually identical. The people who suffered from hyperventilation to the extent that it was obvious – 'the tip of the iceberg' – were very much in the minority.

Dr Lum questioned the practice of labelling patients with over-breathing or hyperventilation as suffering from an 'anxiety state'. 'Anxiety, in my experience, has usually been the product, not the prime cause,' he maintained. Just like Professor Buteyko, Dr Lum viewed hyperventilation as the *cause* and anxiety as the *result* of over-breathing. Dr Lum regarded over-breathing simply as a 'bad habit' that changed the body chemistry and set off a chain reaction, leading to numerous apparently unrelated symptoms.[9] These symptoms, he claimed, may affect any part of the body, and any organ or any system. Similar to Professor Buteyko's findings, Dr Lum claimed these symptoms were reproducible, just by getting people to hyperventilate.

A WORD OF CAUTION

Do not try to reproduce symptoms by hyperventilating or
increasing your breathing. It can be extremely hazardous or
even fatal. Over-breathing can cause arteries to constrict and
can reduce blood flow and oxygen to vital organs, such as
the heart and brain, and may lead to angina (chest pain due
to insufficient oxygen to the heart muscle) and arrhythmias
(irregular heart rhythms).

Dr Lum was certainly ahead of his time. It's difficult to believe
that such labelling and disregard for human suffering could be
found in those not so far-off times (the 1960s and 1970s), yet
how far have we come in this supposedly more enlightened era?
While there have been some advances, chronic hyperventilation
is unlikely to take centre stage as a cause or even as a trigger for
numerous apparently unrelated symptoms.

Sometimes, without even an assessment of their breathing
pattern, people are told they are suffering from 'anxiety' or
'panic disorder'. People who experience anxiety are sometimes
advised to 'relax and take deep breaths'. And, sadly, I have found
that there is still an aura of shame and embarrassment and even
stigma associated with anxiety and panic disorder. Currently,
the key role that hyperventilation plays in patients with stress,
anxiety and panic symptoms is largely unrecognised, or is not
considered important, while medication and talk therapies for
these conditions are given prominence.

Although there are numerous self-help books written on
anxiety and panic disorder, hyperventilation is usually referred

to only in passing, if at all, and the main thrust of the discussion tends to be centred on relaxation or cognitive behavioural therapy.

Breathing retraining techniques may be outside their scope of expertise, but many doctors and dentists are becoming more interested in finding out about them and some may recommend that a patient does a breathing retraining course. As there have now been several studies on the Buteyko method for asthma, many doctors are becoming more familiar with the concept and will most likely respond positively with 'I've had some of my asthma patients do very well with the Buteyko method' if asked about the topic by people with asthma. Nowadays there are quite a few doctors and psychologists who are open-minded about breathing retraining and, in fact, I have taught breathing retraining to doctors and psychologists and given presentations to doctors and dentists on the subject of breathing retraining. Also, I encourage clients to consult their doctor and I like to liaise with my clients' doctors and forward written reports showing patients' pre- and post-course results.

Dentists and orthodontists are also becoming increasingly aware of the issues associated with mouth-breathing and the detrimental effects of mouth-breathing on jaw development in children. (See also the Try This box overleaf.)

During the 1990s, stress and anxiety expert Professor Robert Fried became recognised for his work on hyperventilation. 'Hyperventilation is probably the most common of the stress-related breathing disorders,' Professor Fried maintains, and various reports state that its frequency ranges between 10 per cent and 25 per cent in the general population.[10] There are several medical reports suggesting that hyperventilation causes arterial blood vessels in the heart and brain to constrict, seriously impairing blood flow to these organs, Professor Fried states. He quotes the late Dr H E Walker, a clinical professor of psychiatry, who said, 'hyperventilation is one of the most misunderstood and most frequently overlooked illnesses in medicine'.[11]

TRY THIS

Open your mouth wide (assuming you are on your own, in the privacy of your home). Notice the placement of your tongue. It drops to the back of the mouth. This is why mouth-breathing is not good for children's jaw and teeth development. The tip of the tongue should rest gently forward in the mouth behind the upper teeth when the mouth is closed.

The tongue and the pressure it exerts are vital to the correct development of the jaw and the formation of the teeth. With habitual mouth-breathing, a child's upper jaw may develop into a narrow V shape and may become highly arched into the nasal cavity. When the mouth is constantly open due to mouth-breathing and the tongue drops backwards, orthodontic problems such as crowding and misalignment of teeth may occur. Another factor is that highly processed food is easier to chew and may have a detrimental impact on jaw and teeth development in young children.

Unfortunately over-breathing or hyperventilation remains misunderstood and overlooked even today when we have more scientific ways of assessing and monitoring the breathing pattern. As Professor Buteyko and Dr Lum maintained, once the habit of over-breathing is established, it is the over-breathing that triggers anxiety and panic, not the other way round. In my practice I have seen anxiety and panic symptoms eliminated in just a short time following breathing retraining, and in a later chapter we will take a closer look at these results.

Talking to your doctor or counsellor

Breathing retraining should form a key part of any healthcare management approach to stress, anxiety and panic symptoms. However, if you have issues with unresolved conflicts in your life, I also recommend seeing a counsellor. This will allow you to talk about these issues in private and may be helpful in taking the pressure off.

When you are feeling stressed and fatigued and possibly not sleeping well, your concentration levels may be poor, your head may be a little spaced or foggy and you may be experiencing anxiety or having panic attacks. Under these circumstances, the last thing you may feel like doing is talking to anyone. You may keep hoping that one day you will wake up and the feelings will have gone away. You may even feel a little intimidated about talking it over with your doctor or feeling a little guilty or uneasy that you may be doing something to initiate your symptoms. However, the symptoms are very unlikely to go away without effective healthcare management. And I can reassure you that you are not weak and you are not consciously doing anything to provoke the symptoms.

You are not alone. Large numbers of people experience stress, anxiety or panic symptoms, so your doctor will be very familiar with your symptoms. However, they will not necessarily be familiar with over-breathing as a cause or a trigger for symptoms, or agree that this is likely; your doctor will most likely attribute the over-breathing (if it is diagnosed) to stress and anxiety – not the other way round – and, therefore, may view the anxiety as the prime objective for medical treatment, not the dysfunctional breathing pattern.

It's a chicken-and-egg situation: which came first, the stress, the over-breathing pattern or the anxiety and panic symptoms? Most of us are not born over-breathing, therefore I tend to think the stress came first and triggered the over-breathing, and this in turn triggered the anxiety and panic symptoms. Over-breathing then became a habit, increasing the stress levels and leading to anxiety and panic. In reality, once the over-breathing becomes a habit, there may be a cycle of one feeding into the other, thereby perpetuating the symptoms as discussed in Chapter 2.

As my client Sarah discovered, talking about your issues with trusted friends or family can be very liberating and take a huge burden off your shoulders.

CHAPTER 8

Why am I over-breathing?

Over-breathing triggers

Karen has three young children. She acknowledges that she is a perfectionist and likes everything to be done in a disciplined and orderly way. Like most mothers, Karen finds caring for young children and running a home stressful and demanding at times. Life is often chaotic and the demands of looking after young children and keeping everything in order and up to her high standards are challenging to say the least.

Karen says she has experienced anxiety since childhood and can't really remember when it started. Then she started to have panic attacks when her children were very young. She started sleeping poorly, was waking at night and had difficulty getting back to sleep. With Karen's attacks came tingling in her fingers (as is common in panic attacks) and she felt very drained and shaken afterwards.

So Karen saw her doctor for a check-up, but tests showed no abnormality. Karen tried counselling, which she said didn't help, and she also tried taking anti-anxiety medication for a few weeks. But Karen says she didn't like taking the medication and found it didn't agree with her.

On the day Karen came to see me, she said she was having a good day. But despite feeling okay, Karen's capnometry assessment indicated that she was moderately over-breathing. Karen's respiration rate per minute was within the normal ranges but her breathing pattern was quite irregular. Although Karen was mainly nose-breathing, it was obvious that her breathing pattern was disordered.

Like many clients, Karen had some ups and downs during her breathing retraining course. I advised her to take things slowly. By the time she attended a follow-up review two weeks after the course, her breathing pattern had improved and Karen seemed much more relaxed. She reported that she was beginning to recognise her over-breathing triggers and to take action, as I had advised, to calm her breathing down to prevent the panic attacks from happening – hence the number of panic attacks was considerably reduced. However, at this stage Karen's end-tidal carbon dioxide levels were not yet quite within the normal range and her breathing retraining exercises needed to be continued.

One month after her course, Karen attended for a further follow-up review. She appeared happy and had continued to improve. The good news was that she had not had any further panic attacks; she was sleeping well and rated her sleep 7 out of 10. Karen's breathing assessment now showed that her end-tidal carbon dioxide levels were within the normal range.

Perhaps you discovered from your breathing questionnaire that you may be over-breathing. The next question I am usually asked is, 'Why me? What have I done to deserve anxiety or panic attacks?' Or, more simply: 'Why am I over-breathing?'

No-one 'deserves' to have anxiety or panic attacks. There are several potential triggers and causes that may be associated with over-breathing, including (in no particular order):

- increased stress levels
- emotions (negative and positive)
- possibly genetics
- misinformation about the merits of deep breathing
- thinking that mouth-breathing is better (some western forms of practices such as yoga and meditation encourage mouth-breathing)
- food and lifestyle choices (e.g. sedentary lifestyle, poor food choices, over-eating, eating excessive amounts of animal protein)
- sleeping too much, particularly while lying on the back
- overheated and stuffy rooms
- habit.

Strange as it may sound, the most common reason for chronic over-breathing is simply habit. As mentioned, most of us are not born over-breathing. The habit of over-breathing was most likely initiated by some form of stress from either physical or emotional stressors − or both − and then over time the over-breathing pattern became established and reinforced, without the person even being aware of it. Many people who over-breathe tend to breathe mainly through the mouth, but this is not always the case, as in Karen's story above. Karen was nose-breathing and her respiration rate per minute was within the normal limits, yet her capnometry assessment indicated moderate over-breathing because Karen was taking deeper breaths through her nose.

Some people who over-breathe may predominantly nose-breathe but their breaths may be a little faster or deeper. There may be more subtle clues, such as they take larger breaths when speaking, or they may sigh or yawn fairly frequently, and they may be unaware of this. These are all ways they unconsciously maintain the low carbon dioxide levels they have become accustomed to.

My client Karen's over-breathing was associated with increased stress levels, possibly related to unrealistic expectations, and the body's response to a stressful situation. As Karen admitted, she is a perfectionist. But, as most parents are all too aware, coping with very young children can be hectic and even a little frantic at times. And when we place unrealistic expectations on ourselves, or when others place unrealistic expectations on us, our stress levels increase and breathing patterns change. Karen acknowledged, however, that the stress of caring for young children did not initiate the over-breathing, it merely exacerbated it, as she had experienced anxiety from childhood.

In practice, after I have assessed baseline breathing parameters using capnometry, I request clients to nose-breathe gently. After a few breaths, some clients go from over-breathing with very low end-tidal carbon dioxide levels to normal end-tidal carbon dioxide levels. However, for some people who are over-breathing, nose-breathing for any length of time may be hard to sustain and may even become uncomfortable – they immediately feel as if they are not getting enough air. The habits of over-breathing and mouth-breathing are well established, but this does not mean that these habits cannot be changed – quite the reverse, in fact.

Some clients who experience anxiety and panic symptoms may feel alarmed or even anxious or panicky if they try to sustain gentle nose-breathing that allows for normal levels of carbon dioxide to be retained because they may be sensitive to increased carbon dioxide levels. In people with these reactions, the breathing pattern needs to be improved very gradually, so that they can adapt to normal levels of carbon dioxide and are able to nose-breathe more comfortably.

Shut your mouth and save your life

In the nineteenth century American painter, author and explorer George Catlin travelled North and South America observing the appearance, health and physical condition of the indigenous peoples and comparing these with his own society. Catlin observed striking differences in breathing habits – and in health and physical appearance – between the two, and wrote a book with the rather unusual title *Shut Your Mouth and Save Your Life*.[1]

Catlin reported that the Native American peoples always slept with their mouths closed, and mothers encouraged this habit by gently closing their babies' lips when they put them down to sleep. Due to their habit of nose-breathing, Catlin contended that the Native American peoples had better jaw development and dentition and also did not suffer from some of the diseases endemic among his own people.

The most striking contrast Catlin found was the difference in facial development, such as teeth and jaw development. In his society, people were susceptible to over-crowded and misaligned teeth, whereas the native people had very good dentition and jaw development. Not only did Catlin describe these features, he included several striking illustrations to prove his point.

There may be occasions when mouth-breathing, and therefore over-breathing, just becomes a habit. For example, if a young child has a cold – and of course young children always seem to have lots of colds – the nose becomes blocked and it becomes difficult or even impossible to nose-breathe. Likewise when there are allergies, the child may start to mouth-breathe due to nasal obstruction. The mouth-breathing habit may become established very quickly in babies and young children, and it's possible that they may not revert to nose-breathing once the cold or allergy has cleared. Thumb sucking may be another behaviour that allows mouth-breathing to become a habit, and in addition may lead to poor development of the jaw and dental arch. Mouth-breathing may also be related to the fact that babies tend to copy adults' behaviour. Try sticking your tongue out at a baby and of course they love to copy! If the parents or family members are mouth-breathing, the baby may follow this example and adopt the mouth-breathing habit.

Children who mouth-breathe are more likely to need orthodontic treatment, as the jaw does not develop correctly. Nowadays, savvy dentists and orthodontists are becoming more aware of the detrimental effects of mouth-breathing in children and in adults, and are recommending breathing retraining.

Adults may also start to mouth-breathe due to stress, allergy or nasal obstruction, then the mouth-breathing – and the over-breathing – may become a habit.

In classes, I am no longer surprised to find that children as old as twelve years, and even some adults who mouth-breathe, tend not to blow their noses, and some have never learnt how to blow their noses, which is quite astonishing as it is something most children can manage from around the age of three or four. A gentle reminder and a quick lesson in how to blow their nose may help to change the mouth-breathing habit in young children.

Happy foods and the gut–brain connection

We are beginning to discover how important food and nutrition are – not just for physical health but also for our mental health and sense of wellbeing. From the benefits of the Mediterranean diet to the use of probiotics and beyond, evidence is mounting on how improving the gut–brain interaction may improve our overall physical and mental health.

The information in this section focuses on recent research on diet and includes some cutting-edge research on the gut microbiome in relation to anxiety, depression and irritable bowel syndrome (IBS). Information on these issues was not available in Professor Buteyko's lifetime, although he did advocate moderation in eating and also the use of natural foodstuffs. He also maintained that over-breathing is aggravated by environmental pollution, pesticides and chemicals.

It makes sense that our nutritional intake and our general patterns of eating are directly related to how we feel, our sleep, our mood – and our breathing pattern. When we are stressed and anxious, feeling overwhelmed or under pressure, our digestive system has to try to cope with this added workload as well as digest our food, which is no mean feat.

The gut–brain axis may be the missing
link in several conditions, including
anxiety disorders and depression.

In addition, what and how we eat is critical in helping to balance the trillions of small organisms that inhabit the gut. Studies suggest that there is an important relationship between stress and the gut microbiome. The gut microbiome is the gut ecosystem, which contains trillions of microbiota: organisms or 'bugs' that keep our digestive system running smoothly and help us break down our food so that it can be absorbed. The gut microbiome also forms part of a network called the microbiota-gut-brain axis, or just the gut–brain axis.[2]

Researchers have theorised that the gut–brain axis may be the missing link in several conditions, including anxiety disorders and depression,[3] with the gut microbiome emerging as a key regulator associated with stress and neuroinflammation (an inflamed nervous system).[4] Studies also suggest that the gut (along with the trillions of organisms it contains) is linked not only to our health and mood, but possibly even to the way we think.

This gut–brain axis includes the gut and digestive system, known as the enteric nervous system, which is sometimes called the 'little brain' because of the millions of nerve cells lining the digestive tract.[5] This network links the gut with the central nervous system, the spinal cord and the brain.

Unsurprisingly, the gut–brain axis also links with the autonomic nervous system, which forms a critical part of our response in stress, anxiety and panic. The autonomic nervous system includes:

- The sympathetic division, which governs the fight-or-flight response and increases the heart and breathing rates.
- The parasympathetic division, which regulates the rest-and-digest state, which slows down the heart and breathing rates.

It's only recently that we have begun to realise how profoundly our digestive systems and the foods we eat are linked to our health and wellbeing. While much of the initial research on the gut microbiome has been conducted with animals, there have also been several trials involving humans. Thousands of research articles on the human gut microbiome have appeared in the last decade and hardly a week goes by without another scientific paper on the human gut microbiome. Our emerging understanding on the significance of the gut–brain axis is also linked to a huge scientific project called the Human Microbiome Project (HMP), which commenced in 2008. Key findings from the second phase of this project are still to be revealed as this book comes to publication,[6] and this revolutionary area of research may replace the Human Genome Project as the new frontier in our understanding of healthcare. While the HMP focuses on several areas of the body (even our skin has its own microbiome), a major part of it is concerned with the gut and the trillions of tiny organisms that inhabit our intestines.

Indeed, when it comes to the gut–brain axis the old adage 'you are what you eat' has taken on a new and more scientific meaning.

Other important links are being found between the food we eat and our mental health. An Australian study – aptly called the 'SMILES' trial (the first of its kind) – suggests that eating a

modified Mediterranean-style diet can help to improve anxiety
and even major depression.[7] Researchers found that this diet,
which is rich in vegetables, with moderate consumption of fruit,
an increased consumption of oily fish, legumes (peas, beans and
lentils), raw and unsalted nuts and seeds, extra virgin olive oil as
the main source of fat, moderate consumption of lean red meat
and moderate consumption of reduced-fat dairy products, helped
to reduce anxiety and depression. In essence, this diet is high in
fibre and vitamins (in particular vitamin C), essential fatty acids
and many other vitamins, minerals and essential nutrients that
may be lacking in our standard diet. How could you not love a
diet that encourages you to eat an abundance and diversity of
tasty food as well as providing an opportunity to indulge in a
little wine and some dark chocolate occasionally?

The Mediterranean-style diet is also said to be heart healthy,
lower cholesterol and reduce our risk of cancer, Parkinson's
disease and Alzheimer's disease. For more information, or to
view the Mediterranean food pyramid, see the Mayo Clinic's
website: www.mayoclinic.com.

Why the Mediterranean diet improves health is unclear. It
may be that an abundance of essential fatty acids contained
in fish, nuts and seeds are anti-inflammatory in the gut and
elsewhere in the body. These essential fatty acids (or possibly
other nutrients in the Mediterranean diet) may contribute to
increased levels of serotonin – the 'happy' hormone – in the gut
and the brain. The gut is considered to be our 'second brain' in
terms of producing and storing serotonin, with more than 90 per
cent of this neurotransmitter originating in the gut.[8]

It is quite likely that the Mediterranean diet helps to balance
our gut bugs by increasing the good and starving the bad,

and helps to improve the microbiome through consuming a greater diversity of plant foods, which increases fibre intake. (The SMILES trial mentioned earlier focused on decreases in symptoms of anxiety and depression and not specifically on the microbiome.)

Another factor that suggests a link between the microbiome and mood are the published reviews of randomised controlled trials, which suggest that probiotic supplementation can be beneficial for people experiencing anxiety and depressive symptoms.[9, 10]

The key question is: what does all this have to do with breathing? If improving the gut microbiome improves stress, anxiety and depression, as has been suggested in clinical trials, this in turn may have an impact on breathing via the autonomic nervous system, which is linked to the enteric nervous system and the gut–brain axis.

IBS, anxiety and panic

Many of my clients who experience stress, anxiety and panic also report that they have been diagnosed with irritable bowel syndrome (IBS). Indeed, according to research, there is a strong association between IBS, anxiety and panic. In susceptible people, stress and anxiety may affect the nerves of the bowel, and trigger IBS symptoms.[11]

For decades, IBS was considered a controversial condition and sufferers were told 'it's all in your mind' or 'it's due to anxiety'. We are now learning that this condition – which affects millions of people throughout the world – may not be all in the mind at all, but may in fact be 'all in the gut' as many sufferers have always maintained.

Why the association between anxiety, panic and IBS occurs

remains unclear, despite a great deal of research on the topic. Some researchers have found that IBS *precedes* panic disorder in most people with IBS.[12] However, some people develop IBS and panic disorder at the same time and some develop IBS *after* they develop panic disorder.

Prolonged stress, the use of antibiotics, poor diet and other factors may play a part in reducing the beneficial bacteria in the gut, thereby leading to gut issues and imbalances in the gut microbiome – and potentially to IBS symptoms. The somewhat revolutionary theory that mood and IBS symptoms can be improved simply by eating well and by improving the microbiome – without side effects – is very appealing.

The gut microbiome is generally kept in balance through eating the right foods. When our diet contains excessive sugar, excessive starchy foods and/or too many processed foods and insufficient fibre, our gut microbiome can become unbalanced – a condition called 'dysbiosis' – and we may begin to experience bloating and other gut issues. Indeed, the label of IBS may be a misnomer in these instances, as one of the main criteria for an IBS diagnosis is that there is *no* underlying pathology. IBS is diagnosed by ruling out other conditions and it does not show up on any medical examination or test. Dysbiosis may be viewed as an underlying condition and therefore could negate the IBS label.

With the increasing use of DNA, where researchers can now sequence and identify gut bacteria, as a society we are at the forefront of a revolution in diagnosing and treating gut issues and IBS. A limited number of commercial companies provide this service, but it is expensive and the results need to be interpreted by an expert. Although there is no clear evidence as yet, the fact that the gut and the brain do not appear to communicate as they should in people with IBS may well be due to imbalances in the gut microbiome.

If you have been diagnosed with IBS, you may need to consider improving your gut microbiome through diet and/or probiotics. Consulting a holistic healthcare practitioner who specialises in this area would be helpful. There are also several books available on this topic, some of which are listed in the bibliography.

In summary, however, most adults experiencing anxiety and panic symptoms tend to be very careful about their diet and their nutrition. Many seem to have food intolerances or IBS and are very aware of their diet. Guidelines on food while retraining the breathing pattern are provided in Part 2.

Misinformation and the Deep-Breathing Brigade

We are all susceptible to misinformation on the merits and benefits of deep breathing.

Apart from increased stress levels and habit, the greatest contribution to over-breathing is made by what I term the 'Deep-Breathing Brigade', whose propaganda is frequently seen in the media. These are the people, some of whom may have few qualifications or even no qualifications in breathing, who extol the benefits of deep breathing and advocate deep breathing, with little or no understanding of breathing. Unfortunately, people tend to heed the advice they read or hear in the media and may learn faulty breathing habits, believing that they will get better oxygen levels by breathing more deeply.

People with asthma and people with stress, anxiety and panic symptoms may be advised to 'relax and take deep breaths', but this is not good advice if they are already over-breathing, because it will adversely affect their carbon dioxide levels.

How often are people with asthma or people experiencing stress, anxiety and panic symptoms advised to 'relax and take deep breaths'? Far too often, when we consider that people with these conditions are already over-breathing.

We can all recall being told to 'take nice big breaths in and out through your mouth and puff out that chest! How good does that feel?' The honest answer is, 'Not good!' This is another modern myth promoting the so-called merits of deep breathing. Puffing out the chest does not improve breathing and is counterproductive. In fact, if a person with asthma or stress, anxiety and panic symptoms continues to breathe in this way, they will begin to feel 'spaced out' and dizzy, and if they continue, they may feel faint or they may actually faint.

Puffing out the chest is like blowing up balloons. If you've ever blown up balloons for a child's party, you'll know that after the first two or three you begin to feel a bit off, then after a couple more, you begin to feel nauseated. Blow up a few more and you will begin to feel spaced out and dizzy. These effects are exactly the same as those seen in over-breathing: increases in the volume of air breathed, disturbance of the balance of gases and exhalation of excessive amounts of carbon dioxide. Deep breathing by blowing up balloons does not induce calm or relaxation – quite the opposite – so how could deep breathing help to calm anxiety or panic attacks?

Belly breathing or chest breathing?

If you get the opportunity, observe how a baby breathes. It's called 'belly breathing', which means they are using the diaphragm correctly. As the baby breathes in, its little tummy moves outwards, and as it breathes out, the tummy becomes flatter. This is how we all breathed as infants and it is how we should be breathing as adults – from the abdomen. This mode of breathing is sometimes called 'abdominal breathing'. No air actually enters the abdomen, though, it just appears to enlarge as we breathe in. This breathing is more correctly called 'diaphragmatic' breathing.

The diaphragm is a large dome-shaped organ that separates the chest and the abdominal cavities (not completely: some of the major blood vessels and the oesophagus, or food pipe, pierce the diaphragm). Generally, we don't give much importance to the diaphragm, but it is an essential part of respiration. Basically, as we breathe in, the diaphragm contracts to allow inhalation to occur, then as we exhale, the diaphragm relaxes. By not engaging the diaphragm correctly, due to poor posture or habit, breathing becomes more difficult and can be hard work.

By puffing out the chest as we breathe in, it might appear as if we are getting a larger volume of air and greater lung capacity, but the reverse is actually true. Chest breathing – or 'thoracic' breathing, as it is also known – is a very inefficient way of breathing. Chest breathers usually have to breathe more rapidly in order to achieve an adequate minute volume. When this happens, they are more likely to over-breathe and the habit of over-breathing may then become established.

TRY THIS

Chest or abdominal breathing?

Put one hand flat on your upper chest, roughly in the middle.

Place your other hand flat on your upper abdomen, in the centre, just below your rib cage.

Now take a normal breath in through your nose and notice which hand moves as you breathe in.

If you are breathing from the abdomen, the lower hand will be slightly pushed outwards and move forwards as you breathe in, while the upper hand will hardly move.

If your upper hand is pushed outwards as you breathe in, and the lower hand remains still, this suggests that you are breathing from the chest.

In classes, I caution people about practising or doing too much abdominal or 'belly' breathing. For most people with anxiety and panic symptoms it's hard to do, it feels wrong and it's even harder to sustain. In fact, it's not something I recommend doing, and in practice I find that improving posture as described in Part 2 leads to more effective use of the diaphragm without focusing on belly breathing. People who are not used to abdominal breathing may develop very sore abdominal muscles, as if they have overdone the sit-ups exercise, and they may also begin to over-breathe from the diaphragm, which will not be helpful or healthy.

By now, you will probably realise that 'the art of breathing' (as one of my clients referred to it) is not simple. It's a very complex process and a minor miracle, but one that sustains us throughout life. And even if there are problems, the body — which is a wonderful machine — tries to compensate and keep us safe.

CHAPTER 9

Stressed out and can't relax

Good stress, bad stress

'Is it okay if I stand for a while?' Jeff asked. 'I can't sit down for long; it makes me feel very uncomfortable and I need to walk around.'

I was somewhat taken aback by this request. Jeff is a fit-looking young man in his twenties, who came to my practice for help with stress, anxiety and panic attacks. He had seen his doctor regularly in the preceding months and was receiving counselling. However, Jeff said he was continuing to experience fatigue, anxiety, panic, shortness of breath and sleep difficulties. When Jeff filled in his breathing assessment questionnaire, he ticked the Frequently column for almost every question.

But as our consultation progressed, Jeff seemed to become more and more anxious and restless, and it became evident that his concentration levels were very low. So when he asked if he could stand, I replied that it was fine. In fact, the remainder of our discussion was done while he was moving around. This was something I had never experienced before: here was a young man who was so stressed out he couldn't relax sufficiently to sit down even for a few minutes.

Eventually, Jeff did sit down long enough for his capnometry assessment and it was not surprising to find that his breathing pattern was very irregular and his end-tidal carbon dioxide levels were significantly reduced, indicating severe to serious over-breathing.

Not only that, his heart rate was over 100 (the normal resting adult heart rate is around 50–80 beats per minute) and his heart rhythm was also irregular. Jeff's breathing rate was almost 30 breaths per minute and irregular (the optimal breathing rate is 8–14 breaths per minute for an adult). No wonder Jeff was having so many health issues.

Jeff's breathing pattern and his symptoms gradually improved during the breathing retraining course and he seemed far more relaxed when he attended for his follow-up review a couple of weeks later. He said he was sleeping much better and feeling well, and that most of his symptoms had been eliminated. His capnometry review this time showed a very different picture from his initial assessment. Jeff's end-tidal carbon dioxide levels were not only improved, they were now in the optimal range. In addition, Jeff's breathing and heart rates had improved and were now regular and within the normal ranges.

And, finally, Jeff had no trouble sitting down for as long as he wanted without feeling uncomfortable or restless.

Stress. It can affect our physical and mental health, and can rob us of sleep, vitality and wellbeing. As we can see from Jeff's story – and others in this book – mental health and physical health are inextricably linked; it's impossible to separate one from the other. We've all experienced increased stress levels from time to time. Work, study, making a living, financial issues, health issues and keeping up with commitments all take their toll. Unlike our ancestors, who had the support of an extended family or even a tribe, many of us no longer have the benefit of family support. Nowadays our families and relatives (our tribe, in hunter-gatherer terms) may live in another city or even in a different country or continent. Many of us are forced to be independent and self-reliant without the benefits of an extended family. The tough examination, the important job interview and challenging life events such as trauma or bereavement are just some of the stresses we may have to face. Combine this mix with our indoor lifestyle,[1] noise, pollution and traffic, and our stress levels markedly increase until we feel overwhelmed. And in recent years 'tree change', 'sea change' and 'downsize' have all become part of our vocabulary in our efforts to combat stress.

Good stress, bad stress

We all need a little stress in our lives now and then. It helps us to get out of our comfort zone, overcome challenges and feel good about ourselves. Some people thrive on stress and actively seek it out. The athlete who competes, the public speaker or actor in front of an audience, the mountain climber striving for the summit all have to cope with increased stress levels. Some people may be labelled 'adrenaline junkies' or 'thrill seekers' because of their love of stressful situations. Such people benefit physically and emotionally from their 'adrenaline high' and experience a sense of achievement from taking on challenges. But these high-adrenaline stressors are usually short-lived and are very different from the prolonged stresses of modern life.

Stress is the body's response to a stressful event or situation, i.e. a stressor.

I will never forget Jessica, a young woman almost incapacitated by severe asthma attacks and unable to work before enrolling in one of my breathing retraining classes. When I mentioned in class that not all stress is bad stress, Jessica's reaction surprised many of her classmates. 'Tell me about it,' she said. 'I ended up in the emergency department with asthma during my engagement party!' One would think that having a party is a happy time and a way to de-stress, but this is not always the case. The excitement and the emotion involved can lead to increased adrenaline levels, thereby increasing the heart and the breathing rates, and, for someone who is already habitually over-breathing, triggering symptoms.

Incidentally, Jessica came to see me a few years later. She reported that just a few months after her breathing retraining course, she had climbed a very high mountain without having asthma attacks or needing her asthma medication. Her breathing pattern had improved, so her stress levels were no longer affecting her and causing symptoms.

Chronic stress

In fact, some people who experience chronic stress (like my client Jeff) are so accustomed to it, they may not be aware that it's affecting their health. We have all interacted with people who are tightly wound, yet if you ask them if they are okay, they will insist that they are fine. Over time the body can adapt and compensate for stress, without the person even realising it – but there may be health consequences in the long term.

Stress has a powerful effect on the body and mind. When stress is so severe or prolonged that the symptoms are disrupting our ability to cope with life, we need to find ways to improve our adaptability to stress, or even to seek professional counselling.

As previously discussed, the fight-or-flight response is activated in stressful situations. When we perceive a threat to our welfare, the powerful stress hormones adrenaline and cortisol are released. Unfortunately, nowadays life can be very stressful and for some people the stress response can become activated on a daily basis. The levels of these stress hormones, along with other stress-related chemicals that help us to fight infection, may increase and stay elevated for longer periods.[2]

Adrenaline increases may lead to:

- An elevated heart and breathing rate, and increased blood flow to muscles.
- Energy requirements increasing, such as when sugar stores (glycogen) from the liver are released and used as glucose.
- Insulin levels increasing in order to allow us to use glucose for energy to fight or run away.
- Low blood sugar levels (hypoglycaemia) developing when glucose stores are used up, which in turn increase the feelings of nervousness, shaking, anxiety, or light-headedness.

These reactions are all identical to those discussed in the section about panic attacks.

Cortisol is a hormone that is produced not only in response to physical trauma or prolonged stress but also in association with rewards and pleasure, for example food and sex.[3] Cortisol at normal levels is actually anti-stress, anti-inflammatory and in addition regulates metabolism (food absorption and energy production) and immune function. Cortisol within the normal ranges is a good thing. However, increased cortisol levels due to prolonged stress or trauma can cause problems. High cortisol levels may impact on sleep, causing insomnia or waking at night, and as a consequence sleep is not refreshing.

Cortisol levels may be increased in 'burnout', which is a condition where someone is physically and mentally exhausted and finds it very difficult to cope with everyday life. In fact, when stress is prolonged, high cortisol levels may also be associated with compromised or decreased immune function, which may lead to increased infections such as colds and flu. Decreased immune function may also be associated with the development of cancer and autoimmune disease.

The high levels of cortisol induced by stress may also be associated with weight gain. Studies suggest that animals gain weight when they are stressed, even when they are eating the same number of calories as when they are not stressed. The body may perceive that stress – whether due to emotional conflict or to physical trauma – may potentially be related to something that is critical to our survival or could lead to our extinction, therefore we lay down extra stores of fat, just in case there is a famine. It was this ability to put on weight and store fat that enabled early humans to survive in cold, hostile conditions or on a long trek in search of food.[4]

While some people may gain weight when stressed, others may lose weight. As I mentioned, in my practice I have found that people experiencing anxiety and panic symptoms are generally very careful about their nutrition, although if they are severely stressed they may not have the energy to organise meals or to be bothered about adequate nutrition. In some instances they may even lose weight due to loss of appetite.

The effects of stress, anxiety and panic symptoms can be far-reaching and, for some people, may have a tremendous impact on quality of life and on the capacity to cope with everyday life.

FIGURE 9.1: EFFECTS OF STRESS

- Anxiety
- Changes in hormone levels
- Anger/irritability
- Stomach upset
- Tiredness/fatigue
- Headache
- Muscle pain
- Insomnia
- Difficulty in getting to sleep
- Un-refreshing/poor sleep
- Semi-waking/waking at night
- Reduced concentration levels
- Reduced work performance (can't concentrate, low energy)
- Burnout
- Poor quality of life
- Reduced immune function
- Mood changes
- Changes in sex drive
- Depression
- Weight gain or weight loss
- Loss of confidence
- Drug or alcohol abuse

Figure 9.1 lists some of the potential effects of stress and is fairly lengthy, but thankfully not everyone will have all of these symptoms or conditions, particularly if the stress is not significant or prolonged and early stress intervention is initiated.

My client Jeff's story is a classic example of the association between stress and chronic over-breathing. Like many of my clients, Jeff's over-breathing and stress levels had gradually increased over time and led to sleep problems, fatigue and a multitude of seemingly unrelated symptoms.

So why did Jeff find it difficult to sit down? Although he didn't realise it, by walking around Jeff was intuitively trying to improve his breathing pattern and calm himself down. By walking around, Jeff was probably:

- Simulating fleeing and thereby reducing the adrenaline surges created by the fight-or-flight response.
- Reacting to adrenaline surges and as a result becoming hypervigilant – on the lookout for danger.
- Attempting to increase his carbon dioxide levels. When we increase energy levels by exercising, moving around or walking, we also increase carbon dioxide levels temporarily.

In Jeff's case, it is likely that his restlessness was partly his body's attempt to try to increase his carbon dioxide levels towards normal and thereby improve his breathing pattern and reduce his anxiety.

Figure 9.2 shows how the hormones adrenaline and cortisol are associated with stress and illustrates how habitual and prolonged over-breathing may contribute to the development of other symptoms. One symptom may feed into the other, increasing the breathing pattern and causing and perpetuating symptoms. Stress-induced over-breathing leads to a lowering of carbon dioxide levels in the body (in medical terms, this is referred to as a carbon dioxide deficit, or 'hypocapnoea'). Prolonged over-breathing and exhalation of excessive amounts of carbon dioxide may lead to the development of several symptoms and conditions, depending on the duration and the degree of the stress, and the severity of the over-breathing. Not everyone develops panic attacks, but stress and anxiety go hand in hand and the two are usually associated.

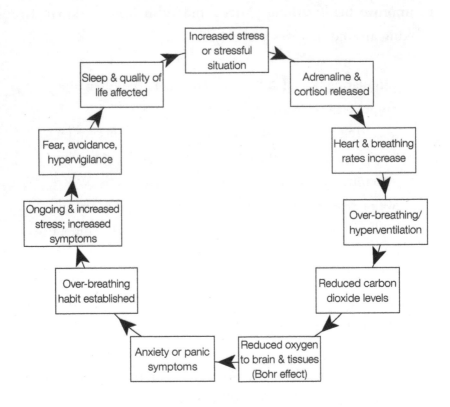

Figure 9.2: Stress, hormones, over-breathing and increasing symptoms

Reduced carbon dioxide levels are associated with changes in blood chemistry and increased alkalinity in the blood. Depending on the severity and the duration of the over-breathing, this reduction in carbon dioxide levels may cause a cascade of other symptoms and changes such as:

- narrowing of blood vessels (vasoconstriction)
- reduced oxygen to the brain (cerebral hypoxia)
- reduced glucose to the brain cells as a result of constriction or narrowing of the blood vessels
- increased stress levels, therefore increasing anxiety and panic symptoms
- a condition called 'hypervigilance' or being constantly on high alert.

How we survive – without having to think

The most complicated and most fascinating system in the body is, I believe, the nervous system. It's so complex that most of us would not lay claim to understanding all of it or even a tiny part of it.

Two of our survival systems already mentioned are the autonomic nervous system (ANS) and the limbic system. Both of these systems could be said to be the body's automatic back-up systems in times of emergency and help us to survive, sometimes without having to think or analyse the situation. The ANS is constantly active and regulates breathing, heart rate and metabolic processes. This involuntary or unconscious control is achieved via two of its divisions, the sympathetic nervous system and the parasympathetic nervous system. (It was called the 'autonomic' nervous system because it was thought that this system was entirely self-governing, but we now know that certain activities can help to consciously calm down the breathing and heart rates.[5])

The sympathetic division increases breathing and heart rates and is associated with the fight-or-flight response, while the parasympathetic division slows the heart rate and the breathing rate down and is concerned with relaxation and calmness – sometimes called 'rest and digest'.

You may have heard of 'sympathetic dominant' individuals, whose sympathetic nervous systems are said to be on high alert, which is thought to make them more prone to anxiety, increased heart and breathing rates, and more susceptible to the effects of stress. When stress is increased and over-breathing becomes a habit, this can lead to a heightened sense of awareness or arousal, which means that there may be a hair-line trigger for anxiety and panic symptoms. However, there is no evidence per se for sympathetic dominance. It may be that chronic over-breathing is actually the issue. The sympathetic nervous system and the parasympathetic nervous system divisions are complementary rather than opposed.

The importance of these well-honed survival systems were brought home to me some years ago while driving along a section of a busy one-way highway. I was driving in the fast lane (well, not that fast, around 70 or 80 kilometres per hour), when the car just ahead of me suddenly swerved to the left. I only had time to think, 'He could have indicated', when I saw the blue blur of a car heading straight towards me – travelling in the wrong direction. I did not even consider checking the mirrors or analysing the situation; with a scream, I swung the steering wheel to the left as fast as I could, and the blue car steamed straight on, stopping on the verge some distance behind me. They probably realised they were driving in the wrong direction after two head-on near-misses, but I'll never know what happened. I drove on, shaking and with my heart pounding, to reflect on what might have happened. If I had paused even for a millisecond to try to analyse the situation, I doubt I would have survived.

One other interesting phenomenon is heart rate variability (HRV), the change in heart rate from beat to beat.[6, 7] As we breathe in, our heart rate speeds up slightly to allow for more efficient oxygen uptake and removal of carbon dioxide. Conversely, when we breathe out, the heart rate slows down to allow to us to conserve energy for the heart to pump more efficiently. These changes in heart rate as we breathe in and out are called heart rate variability. This variability is reduced when we become tense and disappears when we become highly anxious, stressed or fearful.[8]

Sometimes we only have to imagine or visualise a stressful scenario and our heart and breathing rates increase as a result. Even more significant is the fact that we don't even have to be consciously aware of previous stress or trauma – our fears and memories are recorded deep in the limbic system, a part of the nervous system that plays a pivotal role in behaviour and is related to survival, memory, emotions and fears.[9]

This was illustrated quite vividly in an incident concerning a friend – let's call her Erica. Erica was chopping some sun-dried tomatoes and cut her finger, which started to bleed fairly profusely. The amount of blood combined with tomato juice made the injury look worse and caused Erica (a nurse) to panic. This panic was out of proportion to the degree of injury, as it was just a small wound, but Erica's stress response went into overdrive and she couldn't figure out or understand the degree of her panic at the time of the injury.

Later, Erica recalled that she had cut her finger rather badly as a child, and when the recent injury occurred, her brain — subconsciously — immediately reverted to the trauma she had experienced as a child, even though she had forgotten all about this earlier incident. So her panic was out of proportion to the degree of injury for a good reason. We are all programmed to learn from our experiences, and fight or escape — and survive.

Trying to calm down one's breathing or heart rate when feeling very anxious or having a panic attack can be extremely difficult — if not impossible — for many people. There are medications available that may help, but for many people these are a temporary approach. For example, the beta-blocker types of medication such as propranolol are sometimes used by musicians and actors prior to going on stage with the aim of decreasing anxiety levels and reducing stage-fright. These medications slow the heart rate — and therefore the breathing rate — and help to calm the person down. For a short time they trick the brain into thinking that all is calm.[10, 11]

An important question therefore is: could deliberately slowing down one's breathing to, say, twelve breaths a minute, induce calmness in people experiencing anxiety and panic attacks?

The answer in general terms is no. In practice, I have found that a small minority of people who are over-breathing may be helped — on a temporary basis — by slowing down the breathing pattern, though not all by any means. Without the other breathing retraining exercises and strategies, this rate of breathing is not sustainable for any length of time in someone who has a habit of constantly breathing more rapidly. The person may start breathing more deeply to compensate, or will quickly revert to faster breathing, as they find it uncomfortable and may feel even more anxious when they slow down their breathing for prolonged periods in this way.

When I use capnometry to monitor clients' breathing patterns – where they breathe while following a graph on the computer screen – and set the number of breaths per minute at ten or twelve, for example, some people say they feel almost instant calmness and some even feel sleepy. Other clients may become very uncomfortable or even anxious when slowing down their breathing in this way and their end-tidal carbon dioxide levels may even *decrease* as a result. Trying to change the breathing pattern in this way is not recommended, and for many people it is not conducive to calm. Therefore, I generally don't recommend counting breaths. However, if it is found to be calming, a couple of minutes of slow, gentle breathing may be helpful as a temporary measure. For healthy breathing to become automatic, one needs to implement a range of measures as described in Part 2 of this book – not just a few minutes of slower breathing.

My client Jeff was severely stressed and obviously exhausted and incapacitated by prolonged and constant over-breathing, and found it necessary to walk around as a way of calming down. But I am not suggesting that prolonged standing, moving or walking around is an appropriate response to stress, anxiety and panic symptoms – quite the reverse, in fact. While physical exercise may help to reduce stress in the short term for some people, it is not entirely effective if the person continues to over-breathe. Over-exercising or prolonged walking in this way may contribute to burnout, and lead to exhaustion. The best response is to improve and correct the over-breathing and also to learn to deal more effectively with stress.

CHAPTER 10

Plenty of oxygen but short of breath ...

What happens when we over-breathe?

'I constantly shallow-breathe and I can never get enough air, no matter how deeply I try to breathe!' This is how Katie described her breathing pattern on the phone when she called to make an appointment. As I later found out, Katie had experienced panic attacks for years, and despite counselling sessions and anti-anxiety medications, she continued to have symptoms.

Although she wasn't aware of it, like many people with panic attacks Katie had a kind of 'sighing' breathing pattern. Every few breaths she would take an audible sigh and she would sometimes end her sentences with a sigh. In addition, Katie said she yawned a lot and sometimes just couldn't stop herself yawning.

Katie did a course of breathing retraining and, much to her surprise, she discovered that her attempts to breathe more deeply and her constant yawning were part of a pattern of chronic over-breathing and were actually contributing to her anxiety and panic symptoms.

The feeling of never being able to take a deep enough breath, always desperately trying to take in more air, and a feeling of air hunger are common in people who over-breathe. It is a description I have heard many times.

It may seem counterintuitive but by gradually reducing and normalising her breathing pattern through the strategies described in breathing retraining classes, Katie managed to eliminate the feeling of not getting enough air and also got rid of the panic attacks.

Most people believe that if we deliberately take deep breaths we will get more oxygen in. This may sound logical but in fact, it is not accurate. Deeper breathing at rest does not give us more oxygen and it may even lead to reduced oxygen levels and a feeling of breathlessness or not being able to inhale sufficient air, particularly if someone is already over-breathing. Why should this be, if we are taking deep breaths or possibly breathing faster and there is plenty of oxygen in the air we are inhaling?

The air we breathe in contains 21 per cent oxygen, and the air we breathe out contains 16 per cent oxygen.[1] That 21 per cent is more than adequate for our needs. In fact, that surplus of oxygen in the air we exhale is sufficient to enable us to help someone else breathe by doing CPR (cardio-pulmonary resuscitation) in an emergency. So unless we are on a very high mountaintop (where air pressure is reduced) or there is a medical condition or emergency where oxygen uptake or distribution are affected, generally we don't lack oxygen. However, when we over-breathe, oxygen is not distributed effectively throughout the body due to a disturbance in the balance of gases, oxygen and carbon dioxide in the lungs and in the blood. Over-breathing (i.e. breathing in more than the physiological norm) leads to less oxygen availability, not more.

Carbon dioxide: not just a waste gas

Understanding the role of carbon dioxide in the body is fundamental to understanding over-breathing and the strategies used to normalise breathing. There are almost negligible levels of carbon dioxide in the air we breathe in: 0.04 per cent to be exact. This inhaled carbon dioxide level is also virtually negligible in terms of our breathing as we produce sufficient carbon dioxide internally as a by-product of energy production within our cells. It is then brought back to the lungs and blown off as we exhale. However, a significant portion of carbon dioxide needs to be retained in the blood, where it plays an important role in vital body processes as shown in Figure 10.1.

FIGURE 10.1: THE ROLE OF CARBON DIOXIDE IN THE BODY

Carbon dioxide:
- Is critical for our survival.
- Triggers breathing.
- Determines the effective release of oxygen from haemoglobin in our red blood cells to cells, tissues and organs (the Bohr effect).
- Regulates electrolyte balance.
- Acts as a vasodilator, which allows blood vessels to dilate as necessary, including the blood vessels to the brain.
- Acts as a smooth muscle relaxant. (Smooth muscle lines our internal organs such as the air tubes, the blood vessels and the intestines, and if carbon dioxide levels become too low, smooth muscle tends to spasm.)
- Acts as a buffer or balance to maintain body chemistry (by altering the pH).

The optimal range of carbon dioxide in the tiny air sacs in the lungs is 5.5–6.5 per cent. When we over-breathe, we blow off excessive amounts of this gas as we exhale. A gradual alkaline reaction then takes place (called respiratory alkalosis), which is then carried through to the blood, and the total blood level of carbon dioxide is also reduced.

Carbon dioxide is often referred to as a waste gas. This is inaccurate: there is no such thing as a waste gas; *everything* in the body has evolved with a purpose. We are all geared towards survival; *nothing* is left to chance. As everyone knows, we cannot survive without sufficient oxygen; we need it to allow our cells to produce energy, so that the body can continue to function effectively, but, equally important, we also need to retain carbon dioxide at the correct levels.

The kidneys also act as a buffer in maintaining homeostasis or balance within the body. The bottom line is that when someone is over-breathing, they may be inhaling generous amounts of oxygen with each breath but they are unable to use the oxygen effectively, due to reduced carbon dioxide levels and the increased alkalinity that occurs.

Reduced oxygen levels may create a feeling of air hunger or shortness of breath, and this prompts the person to breathe more deeply. But, paradoxically, the deeper the breathing becomes, the *less* oxygen reaches the person's cells and this may create a cycle of over-breathing.

You will find that many of the terms related to breathing have a rather unusual ending: '-pnoea'. This comes from the Greek for 'air' or 'breathing' and is pronounced 'neea'. (Pneumatic and pneumonia also come from the same root.) For example:

- Dyspnoea: (pronounced dissneea) meaning difficulty in breathing.
- Apnoea: (pronounced appneea) meaning without breath or to stop breathing.
- Hypocapnoea: (pronounced high-po-cap-neea) meaning reduced carbon dioxide levels when breathing.

In Figure 10.2 hypocapnoea can be seen as the second link in the chain (after over-breathing) leading to reduced oxygen levels and associated anxiety and panic symptoms. We need to retain a certain level of carbon dioxide and thereby maintain blood pH within a narrow range for effective oxygen availability and distribution. Oxygen availability is governed by a phenomenon called the Bohr effect.

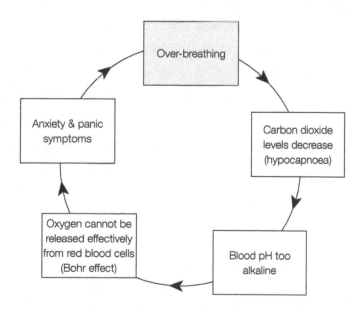

Figure 10.2: Over-breathing and changes in body chemistry

The Bohr effect

The Bohr effect describes how oxygen availability in the body is governed by blood pH. Basically, it means that oxygen splits more readily from the haemoglobin in our red blood cells when the pH remains within a critical level of alkalinity. This scientific phenomenon was discovered by a Danish scientist named Christian Bohr (father of Nobel Prize winner Niels Bohr) in the early twentieth century. It is the Bohr effect that underpins the method of breathing retraining I teach, which is described in Part 2.

When oxygen enters the lungs, it is picked up by the haemoglobin molecule in our red blood cells and is bound to this molecule by a chemical bond. Oxygen is then released from the haemoglobin and distributed to all the cells, tissues and organs in the body through a reduction in the strength of this bond between the haemoglobin and oxygen. The important point is that for this to occur, the pH needs to remain within a fairly narrow range. In other words, it is the blood pH that determines the effective release of oxygen from the haemoglobin. When our carbon dioxide levels are reduced as a result of over-breathing and our chemistry becomes too alkaline, the release of oxygen to the cells, organs and tissues – and to the brain – is compromised, affecting concentration and performance and, ultimately, reducing oxygen levels to the brain.

The Bohr effect determines the effective release of oxygen from the haemoglobin in our red blood cells.

In severe over-breathing, as in a panic attack for instance, oxygen to the brain may be significantly reduced, and as a consequence the person may begin to feel spaced, faint and dizzy. The body will always try to protect itself, and as oxygen levels drop, it goes into survival mode and the person may actually faint, which helps to restore the balance. Faintness, dizziness and confusion that accompany panic attacks are consistent with reduced carbon dioxide levels and reduced oxygen to the brain.[2]

Carbon dioxide sensitivity

In my practice, when capnometry indicates that a client's end-tidal carbon dioxide levels are reduced and their breathing rates are increased, I generally ask them if they would like to try slowing their breathing pattern down a little by breathing with a graphic on the computer screen for a couple of minutes. Some people find this very calming, as their carbon dioxide levels increase towards the normal range as a result of the slower breathing pattern. However, this is not universal. Some people may begin to feel uncomfortable or even anxious with this exercise, at which point we discontinue the exercise. Slowing down breathing in this way does not inevitably lead to carbon dioxide levels within the normal range, as breathing physiology involves much more than the number of breaths per minute. Other important aspects in terms of healthy breathing are tidal volume and minute volume, and these have already been discussed in Chapter 6.

Why some people – but not others – with panic disorder should develop a carbon dioxide sensitivity (where they become anxious when levels increase even towards normal) is unclear. In one small study, levels of 7.5 per cent carbon dioxide gas inhalation over twenty minutes were shown to increase anxiety responses and induce panic symptoms in some patients with generalised anxiety disorder,[3] suggesting that some people with this condition are sensitive to increased carbon dioxide levels.

Therefore, as you will discover in Part 2 of this book, we need to be careful to provide the appropriate breathing retraining exercises to normalise carbon dioxide levels very slowly over time, as going too fast may make some people feel rather uncomfortable or anxious initially.

Why do I have a hunger for air?

Clients with anxiety and panic symptoms frequently say, 'I breathe too shallowly. If only I could take a deep enough breath, I'd be fine.' This is a statement I've heard many times. They feel short of breath, they have difficulty breathing, and they may say that they can't fill their lungs properly or they have a hunger for air. But their capnometry results indicate that they are over-breathing.

> Chronic over-breathing is a condition that may lead to decreased oxygen levels and a feeling of lack of air, or 'air hunger'.

Not being able to take an adequately deep breath and the feeling of air hunger are characteristic of the disordered breathing patterns that occur in many people who over-breathe. In fact, experts theorise that the feeling of not being able to breathe deeply enough may be related to the mechanics of breathing.

We all have some air left in the lungs even after we breathe out, in order to keep the air sacs slightly inflated and to prevent the lungs from totally deflating. This is called the 'residual volume'. Upper chest breathing and over-breathing may be associated with an increased residual volume and, consequently, an over-expanded chest. Therefore, the person may not be able to take a normal volume of air with their next breath and may complain of difficulty in breathing, or 'dyspnoea', to use the medical term.

It can be a very scary feeling when you find you can't get enough air. When this happens, the tendency is to try to take even deeper breaths in an attempt to get rid of that 'hunger for air' feeling and thereby make breathing more comfortable. Trying to take deeper breaths is ineffective, as people with this condition discover, and trying to breathe more deeply may even increase that feeling of air hunger and tightness in the chest and increase symptoms.

By adopting the recommendations and strategies provided in Part 2, you will learn how to retain sufficient carbon dioxide, eliminate that 'hunger for air' feeling and become more comfortable with your breathing.

CHAPTER 11

Sleep issues and over-breathing

Sleep: the great healer

David looked very tired. This wasn't surprising – this young man reported that he woke up several times a night and generally had difficulty getting back to sleep, and this had been happening for years. David had a fairly long list of symptoms, including anxiety and panic attacks, fatigue, low energy and poor concentration. In addition, he said he had palpitations and felt spaced out at times. David had seen his doctor and was on anti-anxiety medication. However, after years of poor sleep, David was exhausted and feeling depressed. David's partner also experienced sleep deprivation because of David's loud snoring when he finally did manage to get some sleep.

Frequent waking at night, as any new parent will acknowledge, is conducive to making anyone feel like a zombie or spaced out the next day. But David did not have children, and there was no obvious reason for his lack of sleep – apart from a disordered breathing pattern and the stress created by years of constant fatigue, anxiety and panic attacks. David's anxiety about waking up and not sleeping well, not being able to study or work effectively the next day, and increasing stress levels had taken their toll.

David's breathing assessment using capnography indicated moderate over-breathing. At the start of the breathing retraining course, David's disordered breathing pattern was most audible while moving and speaking. He was breathing mainly through his mouth, and when speaking he tended to take deep breaths.

Like many of my clients, David yawned excessively at the start of the course, due to a combination of chronic over-breathing and lack of refreshing sleep. But by day five of the course David was no longer waking at night and his self-assessed sleep score had gone from 5 out of 10 to 9 out of 10.

When he attended for a follow-up appointment around three weeks later, David reported that he was sleeping well and that he felt different – he described it as 'calmer'. The panic attacks had gone, the anxiety had improved considerably and his mood had also improved – despite a challenging time at work during this period. The constant yawning was no longer evident. His breathing assessment now showed that he was no longer over-breathing and, in fact, his end-tidal carbon dioxide levels were in the optimal range.

David was happy to continue with the breathing retraining exercises I recommended for a few weeks longer to ensure that his improved breathing pattern remained automatic.

Do you have problems getting adequate and refreshing sleep? Are you tired, tense and edgy during the day but somehow you are not able to sleep well at night? Perhaps you lie awake, mind racing, going over the events of the day or worrying about real or hypothetical situations? Do you have difficulty getting to sleep, or perhaps you wake up and then find it difficult to get back to sleep? These sleep issues are common in people with stress, anxiety and panic disorder. They are also common in people who over-breathe.

There are two distinct issues to consider here: whether sleep is adequate in duration and whether sleep is refreshing. In other words, some people may sleep for ten hours and wake up feeling fatigued and unrefreshed. Others may experience insomnia, have difficulty in getting to sleep, or wake frequently and have trouble getting back to sleep, and of course will be feeling fatigued the next day.

Researchers are finding that refreshing sleep is far more important to health than we once believed – it is as important as adequate nutrition. Lack of refreshing sleep can affect our health and mood, and can make us more prone to anxiety and depression. The bottom line is that long-term sleep deprivation leads to physical, emotional and psychological ill health.

Emerging evidence suggests that disturbed sleep may not just be a symptom of mental health issues – in some instances, it can also be a direct cause. A recent UK study called the OASIS study appears to support the hypothesis that sleep problems are a contributory causal factor in a range of mental health issues, and that improving sleep issues leads to improvements in conditions such as anxiety and depression.[1] In addition, other studies suggest that sleep problems may be a risk for, or even contribute to, the development of some psychiatric health disorders. Mental health issues are significantly more common where there is a history of prolonged sleep deprivation.

The statistics on sleep deprivation and insomnia in relation to mental health are alarming, to say the least. According to the prestigious *Harvard Mental Health Letter*, studies suggest that sleep issues affect more than 50 per cent of adults with generalised anxiety disorder and are also common in panic disorder.[2] Some studies also estimate that 65 to 90 per cent of adults with major depression experience sleep issues. This newsletter further states that studies also suggest that chronic sleep issues affect 50 to 80 per cent of patients in psychiatric practice, compared with 10 to 18 per cent in the general population. Estimates also indicate that poor sleep may be a risk factor for developing an anxiety disorder 27 per cent of the time and may *precede* depression 69 per cent of the time.

Physical and emotional conditions are also common in association with poor sleep. We may be irritable and tired, we can be lacking in energy and make poor judgements, and we may become anti-social and unable to tolerate stress well.

An association between obesity, type 2 diabetes and inadequate sleep has been suspected for some time. Some studies suggest that there may be a link between insulin resistance (a possible precursor to type 2 diabetes) and insufficient sleep in obese adults,[3] but why this occurs is yet to be determined.[4] Weight issues associated with poor sleep may be related to increased cortisol levels, which may be associated with stress. Increased cortisol levels can also be a risk factor for abdominal or central (apple-shaped) obesity, which is linked to cardiovascular conditions and type 2 diabetes.

Health risks of chronic sleep deprivation[5]

People who don't get adequate and/or refreshing sleep are more likely to:

- be obese (particularly visceral or central obesity)
- be irritable
- have lowered concentration levels
- have increased risks for high blood pressure, heart attacks and stroke
- have increased risks for developing type 2 diabetes
- be more prone to motor vehicle accidents
- have increased stress levels
- have lowered immunity and therefore increased infections
- have increased risks for developing psychiatric health disorders.

While the research is still in its infancy, it may be that alterations in metabolism could be linked to how our genes function. One Swedish trial found that even one night of wakefulness may alter how our genes function and that this may explain why shift work can disrupt metabolism.[6] Further studies need to be done but the theory is that processes such as inflammation, immune response and response to stress may be implicated. However, the good news is that gene function can improve and revert to normal expression when sleep improves.

It cannot be overstated: sleep has a *huge* impact on mood, wellbeing and health in general. Most of us are aware of just how awful we feel if we do not get sufficient sleep for prolonged periods of time, but we may not be aware of the full implications for our physical and mental health, and our wellbeing.

How much sleep do we actually need?

It's estimated that adults generally need around seven or eight hours of quality sleep each twenty-four hours. Currently, however, two-thirds of us sleep less than seven hours a night. As my client David found, we can tolerate missing a few nights of quality sleep now and then, but when the sleep debt accrues over months or even years, this takes a huge toll on the body. The body needs adequate sleep to restore itself, rest and repair, relax the muscles and recuperate every night. Sleep is an evolutionary need that has developed over the millennia and has served us well.

Generally, we need to spend around a third of our lives sleeping. That's thirty years if we live to be ninety!

Based on an average of eight hours a night, we need to spend around a third of our lives asleep. But the number of hours of sleep needed is based on individual requirements; some people are perfectly fine with six hours, others may need eight or nine hours to be able to face the day.

In recent years there has even been some debate about the need for an *uninterrupted* period of eight hours' sleep a night, especially from a historical standpoint. In evolutionary terms, did our hunter-gatherer ancestors take it in turns to stay awake and guard the tribe during the night? It would make sense if they did, particularly if there were predators about. A growing body of scientific and historical evidence suggests that expecting eight hours of *continuous* sleep each night may be unrealistic. There is some debate on whether biphasic sleep (sleep broken into two phases) is acceptable and whether or not this was the norm long before electricity was commonly used.[7]

Historically, prolific references exist in literature to 'first and second sleeps', as they are called, in which waking up at night between 'sleeps' was probably considered normal. These references suggest that waking after four hours and pottering about or even socialising and then getting back to sleep for another stretch may not be detrimental and may even have been common practice for our ancestors. But unlike in modern times, our ancestors probably went to sleep shortly after sunset, and then woke up and had a break from sleeping before having what they called their 'second sleep'.

Even today, in some societies where it is very hot during the day, adults and children still take a siesta during the afternoon and are perfectly fine going to bed later.

Modern lifestyles and melatonin

Melatonin is a natural sleep hormone produced in the brain that has had a high profile in the media in recent years. Once the light begins to fade, melatonin production starts to increase and the levels remain high overnight. However, at daybreak, as the sun starts to rise and the light increases, melatonin levels begin to decrease and start to return to a lower daytime level.

How melatonin functions in the body has become clearer in the past few decades. It is thought to be not just a sleep enhancer but also to hold anti-inflammatory and antioxidant qualities. Perhaps there are other qualities which are yet to be identified. Melatonin is produced by the pineal gland in the brain.

Melatonin is a very interesting hormone from an evolutionary viewpoint. It's easy to imagine those happy hunter-gatherers thousands of years ago, sitting by the campfire, becoming more and more drowsy as the light fades and while their melatonin levels start to rise. They fall asleep and stay asleep, courtesy of melatonin. Then – hey presto! – as the sun comes up (no drapes needed) their levels of melatonin begin to drop and they wake.

But it's not so easy for us modern humans. We flood our homes with light as soon as it gets dark and as a result our melatonin levels don't get the chance to increase as they naturally should. Then we use laptops, tablets, smartphones and TVs before bed, which can further reduce melatonin production.[8] A Norwegian study found that reading from a tablet for thirty minutes before going to sleep altered electrical activity in the brain and also altered sleep patterns.[9] People felt less sleepy when reading from an electronic tablet compared with reading a book. The study concluded that the use of tablets may have consequences in terms of alertness and on our sleep cycles or circadian rhythms. Filters that may help to reduce the effects of the blue light of electronic devices are now available.

Excess street lighting may also reduce sleep quality, according to a US study. Researchers interviewed more than 15 000 people and compared their sleep questionnaires with data from a large government meteorological department that measured light radiance via satellite. Higher levels of light were associated with delayed bed- and wake-up times, and there was also a shortening of sleep duration. Perhaps unsurprisingly, people in high-radiance areas were more likely to be dissatisfied with their sleep quality and quantity than people from areas with low radiance.[10]

Snoring and sleep apnoea

Snoring is sometimes thought of as amusing and of very little consequence health-wise, yet prolonged or frequent snoring is a potentially serious condition and may have severe consequences in terms of its impact on health, sleep, relationships and quality of life, not just for the snorer but for their bed partner. Everyone snores from time to time, but excessive snoring is not healthy and can interfere with sleep quality and quantity. In addition, the health risks from frequent snoring may be similar to those mentioned above in relation to sleep deprivation.

One study of people who snore found thickening in the lining of the major arteries to the brain, the carotid arteries, even in the absence of sleep apnoea.[11] Thickening in these arteries may be a precursor for atherosclerosis, or hardening of the arteries, which is associated with high blood pressure, heart attacks and strokes.

Snoring is more common in men, people over forty, and people who are overweight. But it can also affect women and children, and people of normal weight, especially if they mouth-breathe while asleep. Occasionally snoring may be related to nasal blockage due to allergies or viruses. Other conditions such as nasal polyps may be found in relation to more frequent snoring. These are tiny, benign, balloon-like sacs that grow in one or both nostrils and may block the nose. I have had clients report that their polyps reduced in size following breathing retraining.

When snoring is loud and prolonged, the soft palate containing that little dangly bit at the back of the throat, the uvula, may become enlarged and swollen due to the constant vibration and turbulence that occurs during prolonged snoring, especially where there is an increased volume of air inhaled, i.e. over-breathing. This swelling may contribute to the loud night-time noises, and also to a sore throat the next day.

Snoring and over-breathing

Snoring is a sign of over-breathing. Mouth-breathing while sleeping considerably increases the volume of air we breathe in, especially when the person sleeps on their back with their mouth open. It is the excessive volume of air inhaled and exhaled that causes vibration and turbulence and this, combined with a relaxation of the soft palate, causes those loud, raspy noises at the back of the throat.

From clients' enrolment forms I have found that snoring is common in people who over-breathe and it is one of the conditions for which people attend breathing retraining classes. Sometimes the snoring is a problem for the person who snores, as they find they do not get refreshing sleep and they may wake up with a sore throat, headache, a dry mouth or sinus problems. Sometimes the noise from snoring is more of a problem for the bed partner, who cannot get to sleep or is constantly woken by the noise. The bed partner may also experience daytime drowsiness as a result of interrupted sleep. Eventually, the couple may end up sleeping in separate rooms. Repeated nights of disturbed sleep may reduce quality of life and may cause changes in mood or even depression for the snorer – and for the bed partner. Therefore, it's very important to resolve snoring issues.

Although it is possible to snore while lying on the side, snoring and sleep apnoea are more likely to occur while sleeping on the back, with the mouth open and, therefore, inhaling an increased volume of air. When this occurs the tongue moves backwards towards the soft palate at the back of the throat, giving rise to the loud snoring noises or, in extreme cases, to sleep apnoea.

Open your mouth and you will begin to feel your tongue move backwards. Now lie down and open your mouth. It's virtually impossible to keep the tip of your tongue at the front of the mouth just behind the upper teeth. But this is where the tongue is supposed to rest while we sleep, as well as when we are awake.

Sleep apnoea

Obstructive sleep apnoea is potentially a very serious condition and comes under the heading of 'sleep-disordered breathing' (SDB) in medical terminology. It is a condition many of my clients have been diagnosed with before coming to my practice.

Apnoea means to stop breathing. Sleep apnoea is a condition that occurs when a person's breathing is repeatedly obstructed (or partially obstructed) during sleep due to the collapse of the upper airway or soft palate at the back of the throat. The person literally stops breathing for a number of seconds, or even up to a minute. As a result, the person's oxygen levels plummet. Low oxygen levels – or oxygen desaturation, as it is called – may occur several times an hour and possibly hundreds of times a night.

Generally, people with sleep apnoea sleep on their back, breathe through the mouth and snore loudly. They may wake at night (or in the morning) with a dry mouth and feel thirsty, and may need to keep water by the bedside. The upper airway may become swollen and inflamed from the constant irritation caused by air turbulence and vibration as they snore. In addition, they may have sinus problems and headaches. Sleep apnoea signs and symptoms are outlined in Table 11.1.

TABLE 11.1: SLEEP APNOEA SIGNS AND SYMPTOMS		
Stopping or pausing breathing while asleep	Waking at night gasping, snorting or choking	Snoring
Feeling fatigued and/or irritable	Reduced concentration levels	Daytime sleepiness
Sinus problems	Headaches	Dry mouth on waking

Following an apnoea, the person may wake up in panic, sweating and gasping for air or feeling suffocated. Or they may partially wake up hundreds of times per night and return to sleep. They may not even be aware that they have the condition, but they will be feeling sleepy, irritable and fatigued, and most likely lacking in concentration during the daytime. Most people who experience sleep apnoca may say that no matter how much sleep they get, they never awake refreshed. This is because of the reduction in oxygen levels during the constant obstructions in breathing. It may also be associated with the fact that most of the apnoeas or pauses in breathing occur during what is called REM sleep (rapid eye movement or dream sleep), which is an essential part of sleep.

Sleep apnoea needs to be diagnosed by a sleep specialist following a sleep study (which is done either in the home or in a sleep laboratory). The severity of sleep apnoea depends on the number of apnoeas per hour. For mild sleep apnoea, weight loss and diet modification may help if the person is overweight. For mild to moderate sleep apnoea, dental splints (called mandibular advancement devices) may be prescribed. These may help to keep the lower jaw forward while asleep and the mouth closed, which in turn may serve to improve the breathing pattern.

The most common treatment for moderate to severe sleep apnoea is nightly use of a CPAP (constant positive airway pressure) machine, which forces air into the upper airway and 'splints' the airway open while the person sleeps. While it may help some people, CPAP is not well tolerated by around 50 per cent of people, and some may find it invasive and inconvenient. An analysis of several studies in the USA found that 30 to 60 per cent of sleep apnoea patients did not use the CPAP as prescribed.[12]

No-one knows with certainty the cause of sleep apnoea, despite millions (probably billions) of dollars spent in researching the condition. There is a strong suggestion that it is associated with chronic over-breathing, although clinical trials have not yet been done. A survey of breathing retraining practitioners, which I conducted in 2010, suggests significant improvement in several parameters. These include decreased need for appliances such as CPAP machines and oral appliances, and an improvement in sleep quality. Energy levels, restless legs, headaches, snoring and daytime concentration levels also improved when using the Buteyko method for clients with sleep apnoea, according to this practitioner survey. Data obtained from this survey were based on the experiences of Buteyko Institute practitioners and covered more than 11 000 clients with sleep apnoea who had been taught the method.[13, 14] Further, there is other anecdotal evidence that breathing retraining may improve sleep apnoea.[15, 16]

Frequent reductions in oxygen levels combined with sleep deprivation in sleep apnoea increase risk factors for a number of potentially serious conditions. In addition to the health risks of chronic sleep deprivation listed above, a recent analysis of several studies suggests a significant link between sleep disturbances and stroke.[17] Further, recent studies on sleep-disordered breathing suggest that there is a 26 per cent increased risk for cognitive decline in elderly people, meaning memory issues or forgetfulness.[18] High cholesterol levels, increases in blood pressure, heart attack, stroke and type 2 diabetes are also risk factors for people with sleep apnoea. Because of tiredness and reduced concentration levels, there is an increased potential for motor vehicle accidents.

Some research suggests that obesity and obstructive sleep apnoea may form a vicious cycle where each results in worsening of the other.[19] Other research, which may support this theory, suggests that the lowered oxygen levels during apnoea or obstruction may suppress resting energy expenditure (or metabolism) and may lead to obesity.[20] Hormones that signal the brain that the body is hungry, or has had enough food, are ghrelin and leptin. Studies suggest that there is a disturbance in these hormones when there is prolonged sleep deprivation.[21, 22] Ghrelin (think of it as an accelerator) is produced in the stomach and when it is increased due to prolonged sleep deprivation, there is an increase in appetite. Leptin (the brake on our appetite) is produced in the fat cells and helps us feel full. It is decreased when a person is sleep deprived, which leads to a reduction in the signals to the brain that the body has had enough food, and therefore weight gain may occur.

Sleep apnoea is associated with several increased health risks. Quality of life may be significantly reduced and there may be relationship issues, with the couple sleeping in separate bedrooms due to the loud snoring. Anxiety and stress levels may be increased and eventually the person may experience burnout or depression. Therefore, it is very important to obtain a diagnosis and treatment for this condition.

The bottom line is: never compromise on sleep.
Refreshing sleep is vital for our health and wellbeing
and enables us to tolerate stress more readily.

If snoring or sleep apnoea is a problem, you may find that breathing retraining is very effective in relieving or eliminating symptoms, and the strategies suggested in Part 2 may be helpful. However, I recommend finding an accredited breathing retraining practitioner for more targeted, in-depth help for sleep apnoea. Please see the Resources section at the back of this book for details.

As we have seen, refreshing sleep is essential for physical, emotional and mental health. Therefore, one golden rule is: never compromise on sleep. Improving the breathing pattern and sleep enable people to tolerate stress more readily and, therefore, improve quality of life. Better sleep quality has a tremendous impact on stress, anxiety and panic symptoms, as well as improving mood, health and wellbeing. If your partner says, 'You stop breathing at night', or if you find yourself waking up feeling suffocated, or if you are constantly fatigued or experience the symptoms in Table 11.1, you need to consult your doctor for guidance.

In Part 2, we will focus on specific ways to improve sleep, reduce symptoms and increase quality of life.

CHAPTER 12

Avoidance: fear of fear

'I can't go there ...'

Carol is a young woman who had her first panic attack at a shopping centre.

As a result, she avoided that shopping centre and reasoned that if that was the cause of her panic attack, it would be just as easy not to go there and to do her shopping elsewhere. However, the panic attacks continued, and soon there were other no-go areas. By now, Carol was feeling very tense, developing headaches and not sleeping well, and this caused her to feel even more tired and anxious.

Due to her increasing stress levels and lack of sleep, Carol also began to struggle with work, something she had always prided herself on doing well.

Exhausted and at a very low ebb, her world beginning to close in, Carol pondered what to do next. First she visited her doctor, who prescribed medication. This helped to calm her down a little, but the panic attacks were still occurring. She then went for counselling. It felt good to be able to talk about her issues and this helped a little too. But the panic attacks continued.

Carol didn't realise it, but her disordered breathing pattern was impacting on almost every area of her life, from health to sleep, to work and beyond.

Eventually Carol decided to enrol in a course of breathing retraining at my practice. From the capnometer assessment, Carol was found to be moderately over-breathing. As her breathing improved during the course, her symptoms gradually resolved, her sleep improved, and she was able to cope much better with her work.

But Carol realised that she needed to confront her issues, improve her confidence and return to the no-go areas. She decided to do this gradually with the help of family members who accompanied her initially, until she had built up her confidence sufficiently to enter the no-go zones on her own. Knowing that she could control her breathing with the exercises I recommended, Carol felt more confident about confronting her issues, and eventually she was able to return the areas she had been avoiding.

You and your tribe

Imagine you are out in the forest with your tribe many thousands of years ago, happily foraging and gathering food. You are led towards more and more enticing nuts and berries, and suddenly you look around and realise that your tribe has moved on and is out of sight. You are now entirely alone. Then you are suddenly confronted by a different tribe, standing at a distance and carefully scrutinising and watching your every move, and they don't look very friendly ...

Remind you of anything? Stress, anxiety, panic, adrenaline rush – the need to flee? Of course. We survived and flourished as a species for a reason. The human body and the brain have evolved to keep us safe over millions of years, and it is precisely because we use intuition and instinct, as well as logic and analysis, that we have survived. We are perfectly equipped and designed to keep ourselves safe. But at what cost?

Due to stressful events or situations either in childhood or as adults, this survival mechanism sometimes gets out of hand and may become overly sensitive, remaining on high alert. Instead of being an occasional reaction triggered by a potential or actual danger, the fight-or-flight response may become ultra-sensitive. When we look at it from this perspective, the anxiety, stress, hypervigilance and panic attacks for no obvious reason make sense. We may become scared when we perceive something as frightening or potentially dangerous, for example, crossing a bridge, getting lost, flying, overwhelming noises and wide open spaces, to name just a few. All it takes is an association hidden in the amygdala of the brain to trigger the flight-or-fight response. The amygdalae are two almond-shaped structures in the brain related to memory and emotions, and in particular to fear.[1]

Rejection by our 'tribe' (think stressful work situations, relationship or family issues) is still perceived – consciously or subconsciously – as a huge danger: without the help and support of our tribe, we cannot survive.

Many thousands of years ago, when we were hunter-gatherers, getting lost or rejected by our tribe meant certain death. We could not survive for long on our own – and that feeling of needing support persists even in modern humans. Rejection by our 'tribe' (think stressful work situations, relationship or family issues) is still perceived – consciously or subconsciously – as a huge danger: without the help and support of our tribe, we cannot survive.

The body does everything for a reason. Nowadays we are not always part of a 'tribe' in the true meaning, but we need to venture out there into the real world, which we may perceive – consciously or subconsciously – to be full of life-threatening dangers and obstacles. Imagine the actor or the public speaker, the concert pianist, the performer or even the person starting work in a new job. All are out there on their own, away from their tribe, being scrutinised by strangers, just like that hypothetical lone person in the forest thousands of years ago. Is it any wonder that stage-fright is so prevalent and can petrify even the most experienced performers? Or that some surveys have reported that many people would rather die than make a speech in public?

Fear and survival

Like my client Carol, the person with anxiety and panic symptoms may develop no-go zones as their anxiety and panic attacks become worse over time. They develop a fear of inducing panic attacks or increasing anxiety if they venture into certain areas or situations. If, for example, the first panic attack occurred in the supermarket or in the cinema, the person may avoid going there, because the brain interprets that as a potentially unsafe area and sends powerful messages telling them to keep away and avoid that area in future in order to stay safe. Even if rationally we know that the feared area is safe, the subjective and emotional part of the brain sometimes tries to override the rational and analytical part.

Initially, this avoidance may help us to feel safer and more protected, but over time this may lead to increasing issues and a cycle or pattern of avoidance, and the development of further no-go zones as depicted in Figure 12.1.

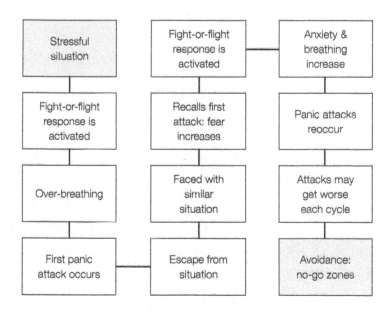

Figure 12.1: Fear of fear: the pattern of stress, fear, over-breathing and avoidance

In its extreme form, the whole world can seem a very unsafe place, and the person may begin to avoid going out alone. This is called agoraphobia, which literally means 'a fear of crowded places'. 'Agora' comes from the Greek, meaning 'place of assembly', and 'phobia' means fear. So while many people love to shop and we even have a term called 'retail therapy', shopping, or even leaving the home, is not at all appealing to people with this condition. In severe cases of agoraphobia the person may become housebound and unable to lead a normal life.

So what is happening here? And why does this fear develop?

Deep in the brain is the limbic system, which includes several structures that have helped us survive for millions of years. This system is still there, trying to keep us safe, even if we're not aware of it. But this survival mechanism can become overwhelmed by stress and fear, and it may start to dominate our rational thoughts.

I am fortunate to have never experienced persistent anxiety or panic attacks. However, many years ago I was on a short flight from Lusaka, the capital of Zambia, to Kitwe, a copper-mining town where I had been working as a nurse at a government hospital for two years. Young and newly married, my husband and I were returning from our wedding and honeymoon in Europe and this was the last leg of the journey. But this was not an ordinary flight. The heat of the tropics ensured that the cabin of the fairly small aeroplane was like a sauna before we even took off. As we reached cruising altitude, the tropical air currents began to cause the worst turbulence I had ever experienced. I don't need to go into detail, but it was a white-knuckles and green-faces experience – I was convinced we were not going to make it and this would be the end of my existence and my wedded bliss before it had even begun! It was a short but significant flight, and I could hardly believe it when we landed safely at Kitwe.

But, as I later discovered, this was to be the start of my fear of flying. I had nearly died (in my mind), therefore air travel wasn't safe. For years I avoided flying and would do anything to get out of it. When my husband suggested a family holiday in Queensland, a three-day trip by road or a four-hour flight away, I would say, 'Let's drive – it's cheaper and we'll see more!' Who was I fooling? If I did agree to fly, it was guaranteed to be a white-knuckle trip for me.

Then I realised that this fear was so inhibiting my life, it had to stop. I decided to confront my fears and flew on holidays instead of going by road. It wasn't easy, I have to confess. I flew to Europe from Australia several times to visit family and friends. In 2000 I even flew on my own from Australia to New Zealand for a conference to meet up with Professor Buteyko. He died around two years later, and if I had not confronted my fear of flying, I would never have met him.

Rationally, I can acknowledge that I am more likely to be killed in a car crash or mowed down while crossing the road than die in an aeroplane, but that emotional and subjective part of the brain perceives that I once nearly died while flying and still wants to keep me away from planes and keep me safe. I try not to allow it to dominate, but I have to confess that I still don't like flying! I practise my breathing exercises on take-off and landing. Turbulence can be unnerving, but nowadays I am not so fearful of flying, nor do I allow that fear to dominate my life as it once did.

Rational versus emotional

We have discussed how the limbic nervous system (which is mostly unconscious) stores memories and fears in order to help us to survive. Small wonder, then, that if we have had a bad experience, such as my very scary flight or my friend Erica's childhood injury described in Chapter 9, the brain tries to protect us – sometimes rather irrationally – from danger. We can see how the pattern and the cycle of no-go zones becomes established as a self-preservation mechanism in Figure 12.1. The fear of fear takes over, which is a mechanism that tries to protect us from harm. This means that the analytical part of the brain, which should be in control, may be overruled by the emotional part, leading to increased fear.

The frontal cortex is the dominant, objective part of the brain, which governs rational and analytical thinking. However, in prolonged anxiety and stress, the limbic system – which may be subjective and governs emotions such as fear and anxiety – is thought to send impulses to the frontal cortex, where they may be consciously experienced as emotions, and therefore the limbic system may begin to dominate.[2] Hence the increased anxiety and fear about entering the no-go zones, sometimes without adequate reason or rationale. Increased stress levels, combined with a fear of fear and a habit of over-breathing, may be all that are needed for avoidance issues to develop. And for Carol, perhaps those high stress levels combined with a highly developed survival system helped to set the stage for avoidance issues.

In summary, there is a direct relationship between stress, over-breathing, panic disorder and the pattern of avoidance. In Part 2, we will discuss how this avoidance cycle can be broken and replaced with more positive memories in order to regain confidence and enjoy life to the fullest again.

CHAPTER 13

How does breathing retraining work?

Research and reality

My client Penny called to give me an update on her progress since her breathing retraining course. Prior to her course, Penny had not been in good health. She had been diagnosed with sleep apnoea but despite treatment, she had continued to have sleep issues and was constantly tired. So she decided to do a course of breathing retraining.

In our telephone update following the course, Penny reported that she was getting the best sleep she'd had in eight years and was feeling much better, which was great news. I advised Penny to have a repeat sleep study done to confirm that her sleep apnoea had improved or had been eliminated.

Penny then asked, 'How can I get through to a family member that this really works? I tried to explain to him that I am so much better, but he thinks I'm very gullible and laughs at me for believing in it.' No wonder Penny was upset. Her relative was struggling with similar sleep issues, and another member of Penny's family also experienced anxiety and panic symptoms. Penny was obviously very keen to help them.

I reassured Penny that all she could do was send them links to the information on breathing retraining for these conditions and then leave it up to them. When they were ready, they would consider breathing retraining. Apart from providing information, there was very little Penny could do.

Penny's story is not uncommon. Most people who do the breathing retraining course are enthusiastic and eager to let family members, colleagues and friends know just how well they are feeling following breathing retraining. 'I know several people who really *need* to do this course,' they say, 'and I can't wait to spread the news!' And sometimes one or two members of the client's family or friends or colleagues subsequently enrol in courses.

But this is not always the case. Some people may think that their condition is different. They may be sceptical or may even be in denial that their breathing pattern is disordered or is linked to their symptoms. In addition, breathing retraining is not like popping a pill, or taking a puff of asthma medication or putting on a CPAP mask for sleep apnoea: people need to be ready to commit to doing the work necessary to improve their breathing pattern. So, I advise clients that when their family or friends are ready, they will enrol. They have to be prepared to do the homework and to commit to changing their breathing pattern.

Attempting to convince someone to improve their breathing pattern may not be a wise decision in some cases, as the person may feel railroaded or may become even more sceptical. When people enrol, all I ask is that they do the exercises with an open mind. I have successfully taught children with asthma as young as four years old, and who of course have no knowledge of science, or why or how the method works. To them it's just a game and we have some fun doing the specific exercises for children.

The Buteyko method

The Buteyko method of breathing retraining has generated much discussion, since it was introduced to the western world in 1990. On the internet, you will find claim and counter-claim about its efficacy. Most of the negative comments appear to have been written by anonymous 'experts' who obviously (from their online comments) do not understand the method or what is involved. Let us look briefly at a few of these claims:

- *The method involves 'hypoventilation' or under-breathing.* This is inaccurate. The method centres on *normalisation* of breathing and a reduction in hyperventilation. The method does not involve *hypo*ventilation.
- *The method involves relaxation, so at best there is a placebo effect.* In other words, the claim is that 'relaxation' is just a sham way of getting people to relax and thereby improve their symptoms. This is something that always makes Buteyko practitioners smile. If we were so good at teaching relaxation, the possibilities in today's stressful world

would be endless! As anyone who has done the course will attest, the truth is that there is very little relaxation involved. Breathing retraining using this method requires a certain amount of work, as well as time and effort on the part of the client.

- **The Buteyko method is not based on science.** This claim is also inaccurate. The method is based on the Bohr effect, which is a scientific phenomenon discovered in 1903 by Danish scientist Christian Bohr, and which is described in most physiology textbooks and also discussed in Chapter 10.

- **There are no clinical trials to show that it works.** This is true for sleep apnoea and anxiety and panic: to date, no trials have been done. The crucial thing here is that several trials of the Buteyko method for asthma show an improvement in breathing pattern, such as a reduction in over-breathing and an improvement in lung function tests, and this is correlated or linked with a reduction in the need for asthma medication. The principles are the same: regardless of the condition, over-breathing is over-breathing and it can be improved.

Health professionals rely on expert analysis such as the Cochrane Reviews to guide treatment.[1] One 2013 expert review from the prestigious Cochrane Collaboration concluded that no credible breathing retraining clinical trials could be considered for review in any modality or discipline for dysfunctional breathing/hyperventilation syndrome, and there was an urgent need for clinical trials in this area.[2] A total of 496 records were screened and were deemed ineligible and excluded – apart from one Dutch trial, which was later discounted as it did not contain sufficient data. This expert review considered including several types of breathing retraining, such as progressive relaxation therapy, yoga breathing, diaphragmatic breathing, biofeedback, and Buteyko breathing. But, as far as I am aware, no trials of the Buteyko method have been conducted for anxiety and panic disorders or for hyperventilation syndrome and, therefore, there were none available for consideration by this expert review.

According to the experts, there is a paucity of credible randomised controlled clinical trials for all methods of breathing retraining for dysfunctional breathing or hyperventilation syndrome. By 'credible' the experts mean that, among other criteria, one group in the trial uses the 'active' intervention – in this case, breathing retraining – and the other group does nothing or uses a placebo intervention known not to change the breathing pattern or symptoms.

While I agree that credible clinical trials are deemed the gold standard in terms of proving or disproving the effectiveness of a therapy, it would be unfair to ask people experiencing anxiety or panic symptoms to wait years until several trials have been conducted. The lack of clinical trials using this method does not prove that the Buteyko method of breathing retraining is not effective, only that the appropriate trials have not be done.

In any event, nowadays it would be virtually impossible to do a 'blinded' clinical trial of the Buteyko method (where the participants are not aware which intervention they are receiving) due to the fact that Buteyko practitioners' information is freely available on websites and it would, therefore, be obvious to participants which intervention they were actually receiving.

And indeed, the inability to blind participants and researchers to these types of intervention is acknowledged by the Cochrane Review authors.[3]

Breathing retraining is not just a useful adjunct or helper; it can be critical in addressing symptoms and in breaking the cycle of over-breathing in anxiety and panic symptoms. Thanks to the internet, more and more people are becoming aware of the benefits of breathing retraining, and not just for asthma.

From an anecdotal survey I conducted in 2012, there are thousands of instances where the Buteyko method has helped clients with sleep apnoea.[4] In addition, there are now several clinical trials and studies suggesting that breathing retraining is effective in asthma. (For further details on asthma trials, please see the section on asthma publications at the end of the book.)

The Buteyko method has been taught to
thousands of people in Australia since
it was first introduced in 1990.

This book is aimed specifically at stress, anxiety and panic attacks and does not contain all the information required for breathing retraining in asthma.

According to a joint Asthma Australia/Beyond Blue factsheet, anxiety and depression are common in people with asthma.[5] This may be due to the fact that people with asthma can become anxious and fearful about having another asthma attack. Perhaps even more importantly, could it be that over-breathing is contributing to or causing their anxiety *and* their asthma?

Several studies of the Buteyko method indicate that people with asthma are significantly over-breathing.

Clients experiencing anxiety and panic symptoms have often had symptoms for a long time and may have tried several approaches to improving their symptoms, with limited or no success. Naturally they may be sceptical and have questions about breathing retraining. People are usually keen to know the science underpinning the method of breathing retraining and, of course, they would like to know the success rates.

So why isn't this form of breathing retraining that I teach being shouted from the rooftops, if it is so effective (even anecdotally) for people with anxiety and panic symptoms? It may be that breathing retraining as a discipline is still in its early stages and is often overlooked, while medication or counselling take centre stage. Or it may be that chronic over-breathing may not be regarded as relevant or significant and, therefore, the emphasis is placed on changing people's thinking using cognitive behavioural therapy, or endeavouring to get people to relax through the use of medication or relaxation exercises. As I have discovered from my clients, these approaches are not always successful.

The main issue, however, is the lack of appropriate clinical trials of breathing retraining for anxiety and panic disorders. To conduct a randomised controlled trial, which is considered the gold standard and which is credible and acceptable to the experts, is both time-consuming and expensive. So the lack of credible clinical trials for this modality is most likely due to a lack of funding.

I hope I am wrong, but I think it is unlikely that there will be trials of breathing retraining for these conditions in the near future. One would not expect the pharmaceutical industry to sponsor a trial on a method that does not involve selling medications! So who would be likely to invest millions of dollars in trials of a method that, unlike medication, would be difficult to patent and has very limited profit-making potential?

Also, when conducting a meta-analysis, or a review of several trials, one has to compare like with like, which is difficult where breathing retraining, or 'breathing training' (as it's sometimes called), is concerned. As well as the Buteyko method there are numerous types of breathing retraining, including several kinds of deep breathing, meditation, guided imagery, relaxation, physiotherapy and yoga, to name just a few. These are all based on different approaches, therefore results will vary considerably. It's a bit like comparing apples with oranges. In some reviews, these methods may be combined as one entity, which will not provide an accurate assessment of their benefits or merits.

Who would be likely to invest millions of dollars in trials of a method that, unlike medication, would be difficult to patent and has very limited profit-making potential?

Several clinical trials in the past twenty years have shown that breathing retraining using the Buteyko method can improve and normalise the breathing pattern in people with asthma. Asthma is the condition for which the Buteyko method was most commonly used when it was first introduced to Australia, and the first clinical trial of the method in the western world was held in Brisbane, Australia, in the mid-1990s, with the findings published in 1998.[6] Since 1998, other studies using the Buteyko method for asthma have indicated that two of the scientific ways to assess the breathing pattern, i.e. end-tidal carbon dioxide levels and minute volume, improved during clinical trials. Some trials only conducted one of these breathing tests, either minute volume *or* end-tidal carbon dioxide levels, possibly because of the expense involved.

We can examine some of the trials for asthma to determine improvements in breathing pattern in this group who undertook breathing retraining. For example, in the first clinical trial of the Buteyko method for asthma outside of the USSR, patients who used this method were found to be over-breathing and their minute volume was significantly increased. The normal adult minute volume is 4 to 6 litres per minute, yet the people who took part in this trial were breathing on average 14 litres per minute at the start of this three-month trial – around three times the normal level. By the end of the trial, they were breathing approximately 9.6 litres per minute and, in fact, this reduction in their minute volume was linked to a reduction in their need for asthma medication.[7] The use of reliever types of medication was reduced on average by 96 per cent. There was no improvement in the minute volume in the control group of people with asthma on this trial who were taught general asthma education and relaxation techniques.

Since then, other studies on the Buteyko method for asthma have also shown improvements in breathing pattern, e.g. improvement in end-tidal carbon dioxide levels[8, 9] as well as improvements in the degree of airway obstruction seen in asthma.[10, 11] If you would like to examine some of the studies related to asthma and over-breathing, these are available online and are listed at the end of this book in the bibliography.

What happens during breathing retraining?

In my practice, breathing retraining courses are generally held over five consecutive days, with a duration of around ninety minutes per day, so it's fairly intensive. Clients put into practice the strategies for breathing awareness, posture, sleep and symptoms learnt in classes. Clients continue to do the exercises and to monitor their symptoms at home and attend my practice for a follow-up review two weeks after their course and again four weeks later, if needed. Courses are generally held in small groups, but individual courses are also available.

What are the success rates for breathing retraining?

Breathing retraining is based on techniques that are used to normalise the breathing pattern. There are a few different techniques around and I can only speak for the method of breathing retraining I teach, which is based on the Buteyko breathing method. We do not refer to it as a 'cure' or a 'remedy' or even as a 'treatment'. Basically, it is an educational approach that is geared towards the individual client, their symptoms and their particular breathing issues. Breathing is very instinctual and, therefore, improving a disordered breathing pattern requires time, effort and patience. However, most people's efforts will be steadily rewarded, even within the first week, with an improvement to or reduction in some of their symptoms.

Clients are often very surprised and delighted at how effective this method is at ameliorating or eliminating symptoms and improving quality of life. Clients are advised to be aware of their breathing pattern and to continue their breathing retraining exercises until certain targets are reached and their improved breathing pattern becomes automatic, which may take several weeks. Course participants are very motivated once they begin to see improvements in their health and wellbeing, often during the first week, and I am often pleased to find that they very quickly develop an awareness of everyone's breathing patterns. They even begin to notice the breathing patterns of their family and friends – and TV presenters!

How long does breathing retraining take?

Breathing retraining takes time. To change something as automatic as breathing takes effort, practice and patience. However, many people will begin to see an improvement in their symptoms and begin to feel better within days, which is a great motivator. Others may take a little longer. Sometimes there are small changes that are not perceptible on a daily basis. That is why I recommend you keep track of your symptoms with the daily diary page and also complete the breathing questionnaire from Chapter 5 before and after your program. You may be surprised how some of your symptoms have vanished – you may even have forgotten about them over time!

As mentioned in earlier chapters, scientific evidence shows that many people with anxiety and panic symptoms are very sensitive to changes in carbon dioxide levels – both increases and decreases – and these changes can induce panic symptoms, particularly when carbon dioxide levels are increased, even within the normal levels. I always assess my clients' breathing patterns before tailoring a program geared towards their needs and their level of sensitivity. So it's a slow process initially, until they become accustomed to higher – though normal – levels of carbon dioxide. That is why it is important to follow the program as set out in Part 2 in order to avoid feeling uncomfortable or anxious, which may occur if you undertake the exercises too rapidly. It would be disappointing to give up prematurely because the strategies recommended were done too soon and made you feel anxious or uncomfortable.

Age limits and breathing retraining

While this book focuses specifically on adults, anxiety and panic attacks do occur in children and in adolescents. Breathing retraining can be done at any age from around four years upwards. I have successfully taught several four-year-olds with asthma, and several people well into their eighties and early nineties. However, the breathing exercises for children are different from those set out in Part 2, and for children I would recommend that you consult an accredited practitioner.

Children and ADHD-type behaviour

In my practice I sometimes see children, usually with asthma and/or who snore, who cannot sit still even for a couple of minutes and who are exhibiting ADHD-type behaviour. Following their breathing retraining course, their behaviour and concentration spans change radically; they become calm and their concentration levels improve considerably. I don't profess to be an expert on this topic, but the obvious question is, 'Why does changing their breathing change their behaviour?'

The story of little Johnnie (not his real name) is worth telling. Johnnie attended a breathing retraining course because of mild asthma. His mother also reported that Johnnie was a frequent and very loud snorer. At six years old, Johnnie was a bundle of non-stop energy who couldn't sit still for more than ten seconds. Six-year-olds are not noted for sitting quietly, but this was different – Johnnie constantly felt the need to move, climb on seats or run around and loudly interrupt with questions, making the class fairly difficult for me, his mother and the other participants. Nothing seemed to calm him down: games, books – we tried everything. Because of his short attention span, Johnnie did not listen to the answers to the questions he asked.

Despite the constant interruptions, Johnnie actually did very well during the first week of breathing retraining and went from mouth-breathing to nose-breathing. When he came back a couple of weeks later for a follow-up review, to my surprise he sat quietly in the chair beside his mother for several minutes, without saying a word, and listened to his mother as she described his progress. After a few minutes of sitting still, Johnnie turned to his mother and quietly said, 'Excuse me,' and went on to ask a question, after which he listened carefully to the answer. This was a different child, and I could hardly believe what I saw!

I have seen this improvement in sleep and concentration repeated many times following breathing retraining courses in children and even in adults, some of whom had been diagnosed with ADHD and had experienced ADHD since childhood.

Could there be a possible association between ADHD and chronic over-breathing, or possibly between ADHD and the lack of refreshing sleep associated with mouth-breathing or over-breathing? I simply don't know. I find it telling that research studies suggest that various sleep problems may affect 25 to 50 per cent of children with ADHD, and that sleep-disordered breathing affects 25 per cent of children with ADHD.[12] There is no doubt that lack of refreshing and restorative sleep contributes to loss of concentration, poor memory and general irritability. This is an area where research is needed.

If a child snores frequently, this is regarded as sleep-disordered breathing and it may lead to unrefreshing sleep: therefore, it may affect concentration levels and daytime behaviour. Sometimes snoring in children may be related to a blocked nose due to allergy or to enlarged adenoids, which are generally associated with mouth-breathing. Accordingly, I would recommend consulting your doctor if your child is snoring frequently. However, I would also recommend breathing retraining before removing enlarged adenoids, as they sometimes shrink if breathing is improved, which may prevent the need for surgery.

CHAPTER 14

Results from my practice

Monitoring the breathing pattern

'I have to put myself first.' This was my client Jenny's somewhat surprising statement during her breathing retraining course.

Jenny was a quiet, thoughtful woman in her forties who enrolled in a breathing retraining course to help her overcome the stress, anxiety and panic attacks she was experiencing. Like many of my clients, Jenny had also been diagnosed with irritable bowel syndrome.

Due to relationship issues, Jenny had separated from her partner after several years together. Jenny realised that the stress caused by the relationship issues had affected her badly and as a result she had developed panic attacks. She decided that for once she had to put herself first, end the relationship and get help for her panic attacks. But the panic attacks persisted even after the relationship ended. And this was why Jenny turned up at my class.

The first step to improving breathing is to develop an awareness of one's breathing pattern. I explained to Jenny that disordered breathing is a habit just like any other, so it's important to be aware of what is going on and how symptoms are linked to breathing, while attempting to improve the breathing pattern.

Jenny's initial breathing assessment using a capnometer showed moderate over-breathing and an irregular breathing pattern. Over the first few days of the course, Jenny realised she was mouth-breathing – and therefore over-breathing – particularly when she felt stressed. Working to improve this habit took some time but it brought rewards.

At her follow-up assessment three weeks later, Jenny seemed much more at ease. Her sleep, which had been poor, had improved. In addition, Jenny said that the IBS was under control. Jenny's breathing pattern had improved significantly and her breathing assessment showed that her end-tidal carbon dioxide levels were in the low normal range. Jenny was delighted to report that she was no longer having panic attacks.

Since 2008, I have been fortunate in being able to monitor my clients' breathing patterns using a capnometer, a non-invasive scientific instrument that measures end-tidal carbon dioxide levels ($ETCO_2$). This type of carbon dioxide measurement is regarded as a reliable and objective indicator of breathing status. As we have discussed, end-tidal carbon dioxide levels are reduced when a person is chronically or intermittently over-breathing.

When we over-breathe, we are not only inhaling an excessive air volume, we are also exhaling excessive amounts of carbon dioxide, and it is the carbon dioxide levels we exhale that are measured using the capnometer. The capnometer I use[1] calculates a number of measurements:

- end-tidal carbon dioxide levels – live and in twenty-second averages
- the breathing pattern in waveform
- the breathing rate – live and in twenty-second averages
- the heart rate – live and in twenty-second averages
- heart rate variability.

My clients are provided with almost instant feedback on their breathing patterns as they can view all of this information on a computer screen. They can see whether their breathing is regular or irregular. They can also see how the effects of posture and the use of the diaphragm, as well as gentle nose-breathing, may impact on their breathing pattern, and on their carbon dioxide levels. In addition, they can observe how a few minutes of relaxation can improve breathing.

This method of monitoring the breathing pattern has provided tremendous insight into breathing patterns for me and my clients, and is especially reassuring for clients with stress, anxiety and panic symptoms. While clients can see how their breathing pattern is disordered, they can also be reassured that with time and practice their carbon dioxide levels can normalise, even if it is only for a few seconds or minutes initially. For my clients, and for myself, this confirms that there is the capacity to improve their breathing pattern.

There is a facility on this instrument to set a lower rate of breathing for the client to adopt and follow. For example, if someone is breathing at a rate of 20 breaths per minute (the optimal adult rate is 8–14 per minute), they may follow a pattern of breathing at, say, 12 or 14 breaths per minute. Some clients may find this calming. However, breathing more slowly in this way does not necessarily improve carbon dioxide levels for everyone. And even for those who feel comfortable in slowing down their breathing pattern, the improvements are temporary. In Part 2 of this book you will discover that a range of strategies and techniques are necessary to improve the breathing pattern.

Capnometry is a very effective tool for monitoring and assessing the breathing pattern while clients retrain their breathing. Some clients find it reassuring to breathe while following a program that allows them to synchronise their breathing with a slightly reduced breathing rate and a regular breathing pattern. I find that an initial breathing assessment using a breathing questionnaire and capnometry assessment before the course and then repeated two weeks after the course (and if needed four weeks later) is sufficient to track improvement.

Results from my practice

As breathing is a dynamic process, all of these capnometry measurements are just a snapshot in time. The capnometer does not show what the breathing pattern is like if the person is under a lot of stress or if they are very anxious or actually having a panic attack – unless, of course, these are happening at the time of the assessment. Nevertheless, these levels provide a very good indication of breathing pattern in general, as I always allow clients time to relax and unwind before their breathing assessment.

Table 14.1 shows capnometry results from before and after breathing retraining courses from a random sample of clients from my practice who enrolled in a breathing retraining course because of stress, anxiety, panic and other symptoms.

In this table, measurements prior to breathing retraining courses show reduced end-tidal carbon dioxide levels in the majority

	SEX	SYMPTOMS/ CONDITIONS	END-TIDAL CO$_2$		RESPIRATION RATE		HEART RATE	
			Before	After	Before	After	Before	After
1	F	Anxiety, stress, shortness of breath	30	38	15	14	90	70
2	M	Anxiety, panic attacks, stress, fatigue, sleep problems	24	40	28	14	104 irregular	80 regular
3	F	Anxiety, stress, migraines	34	37	15	10	70	64
4	F	Panic attacks, sleep problems, shortness of breath	27	33	20 erratic	16 regular	106 irregular	82 regular
5	M	Anxiety, loss of memory, mouth-breathing	34	38	12	15	80	73
6	F	Anxiety, breath holding, mouth-breathing	29	38	14	13	74	72
7	M	Anxiety, panic attacks, stress, sleep problems	37	40	14	13	72	66
8	F	Anxiety, panic attacks, migraines, dizziness	23	31	9	12	78	70
9	M	Anxiety, shortness of breath on exercise	34	45	20	12	88	68
10	M	Anxiety, panic attacks, sleep apnoea	32	41	18	8	72	77
11	M	Anxiety, panic attacks, migraines	33	37	14	18	64	64
12	M	Anxiety, panic attacks, asthma	34	40	20	13	88	73
13	F	Anxiety, panic attacks, insomnia, depression	35	38	12	10	80	70
14	F	Anxiety, panic attacks	27	34	10	7	88	80
15	F	Anxiety, panic attacks, asthma, sleep apnoea	32	37	15	15	78	82
16	M	Panic attacks, sleep issues, stress	27	39	18	14	88	75

TABLE 14.1: BREATHING RETRAINING RESULTS FROM MY PRACTICE (AGE RANGES: EARLY TEENS TO LATE SEVENTIES)

ETCO$_2$ ranges in mmHg:

Higher normal	40–45
Low normal	35–40
Mild to moderate over-breathing	30–35
Serious to moderate over-breathing	25–30
Severe to serious over-breathing	20–25

of clients, which suggest moderate to severe over-breathing. Two clients' (2 and 8) results indicate severe to serious over-breathing. However, ETCO$_2$ levels for another two clients (7 and 13) are within the normal range pre-course. These normal levels may be associated with *intermittent* over-breathing, as these clients subsequently improved their breathing pattern and their symptoms following breathing retraining courses. Results also show that respiration rates and heart rates improved in most clients, including the two clients who had previously shown normal ETCO$_2$ levels.

The after-course results shown in Table 14.1 are taken from clients within two to eight weeks of commencing breathing retraining courses. Clients also kept a daily record of their symptoms and sleep scores. In addition to improved ETCO$_2$ levels, improvements in breathing patterns were also linked to improvements in symptoms (not shown here).

While a capnometer is a useful tool to monitor the breathing pattern, I can also get a very good assessment of breathing status using other methods. From 1999 to 2007 I did not have access to this scientific tool to assess breathing patterns, but my clients still achieved very good results using other methods, including a breathing questionnaire and monitoring their symptoms and results on a daily diary page, combined with a physical assessment of posture and breathing.

Carbon dioxide levels before and after courses

From my practice, I have found that after two to four weeks of breathing retraining, clients' end-tidal carbon levels are generally significantly improved and their symptoms are also improving. Chart 1 depicts pre-course and after-course $ETCO_2$ levels from the same randomly selected clients whose results were shown in Table 14.1.

End-tidal carbon dioxide levels are measured at the end of the stream – or tide – as someone breathes out. Using capnometry, a figure of 35mmHg and above means that the person is breathing within the normal range and is retaining sufficient carbon dioxide and therefore not over-breathing. Below 35mmHg means that the person is exhaling excessive amounts of carbon dioxide and indicates that they are over-breathing.

If you examine Chart 1 carefully, you can see that before their breathing retraining courses, the majority of the clients, except two already mentioned (7 and 13), were over-breathing, with

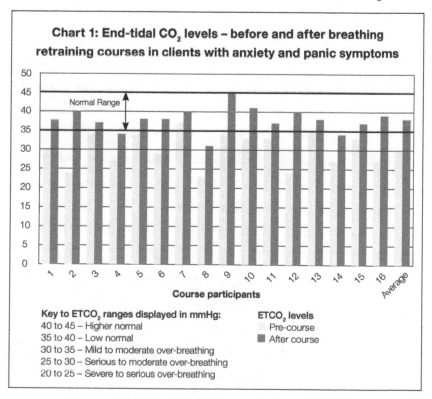

Chart 1: End-tidal CO_2 levels – before and after breathing retraining courses in clients with anxiety and panic symptoms

Course participants

Key to ETCO₂ ranges displayed in mmHg:
40 to 45 – Higher normal
35 to 40 – Low normal
30 to 35 – Mild to moderate over-breathing
25 to 30 – Serious to moderate over-breathing
20 to 25 – Severe to serious over-breathing

ETCO₂ levels
Pre-course
After course

$ETCO_2$ levels indicating moderate to serious over-breathing. At approximately two to eight weeks following the course (this depended on their follow-up review date), all of the clients had improved significantly and the majority of clients were demonstrating $ETCO_2$ levels above 35mmHg, which is within the normal range.

Three clients whose carbon dioxide levels were still below 35mmHg following the course had shown a considerable improvement in their breathing pattern, and although not yet within the normal range, they had improved from severe or serious over-breathing to moderate over-breathing, which is a remarkable achievement within a short timeframe. Clients are advised to continue with the breathing retraining exercises until they reach certain targets and their symptoms are alleviated.

Overall, there is an average improvement in $ETCO_2$ levels from 30mmHg to 38mmHg – well within the normal range – which is a vast change. These improvements in breathing pattern are linked to a reduction in symptoms, which are gradually reduced and eventually eliminated as breathing improves.

For this new and improved pattern of breathing to become automatic, I generally recommend a minimum of four to six weeks of breathing retraining exercises, or even longer in some instances, depending on a client's response.

These results from my practice are anecdotal and are based on a very small sample; they are by no means equivalent to an appropriate clinical trial. From my practice, and from several years of assessing clients' breathing patterns using capnometry and monitoring their symptoms, I am confident that the majority of clients with anxiety and panic symptoms improve significantly using the method of breathing retraining I teach.

I feel privileged to have helped people to make such improvements in their health and wellbeing.

What are the health benefits of improving the breathing pattern?

The benefits of improving the breathing pattern can be physically, mentally and emotionally significant. Chronic over-breathing is extremely tiring and may place a tremendous strain on the heart, lungs and immune system. Being constantly in a state of high alert, or hypervigilance – which is what may occur with stress, anxiety and over-breathing – takes a tremendous toll on all of the systems of the body. This load is lifted quite quickly when we begin to breathe normally again. Increased energy levels and the ability to have a good night's sleep contribute significantly to better self-esteem and improved mood.

Apart from feeling and looking better, there are some unexpected benefits. My clients are sometimes surprised that they can exercise again without getting breathless, often within a few weeks of breathing retraining. And, because they are getting better oxygenation to the heart, brain and tissues, their endurance levels are also improved. The following list shows some of the benefits I have observed in clients who improved their breathing pattern.

HEALTH IMPROVEMENTS FOLLOWING BREATHING RETRAINING

- Ability to nose-breathe comfortably
- Decreased or eliminated anxiety and panic symptoms
- Better self-esteem
- Improved confidence

- Feeling better
- Improved quality of life
- Better mood
- Improved ability to deal with stress
- Better oxygenation
- Improved sleep
- Better concentration levels
- Improved physical endurance
- Increased energy levels
- Increased exercise tolerance
- Physical and emotional symptoms improved or eliminated
- Blood pressure improvements
- Chest pain ceased
- Breathing rate normalised
- Breathing rhythm normalised
- Heart rate normalised
- Palpitations ceased, irregular pulse normalised
- Better circulation
- Improved immune function, fewer colds and flu
- Improved digestion
- Less fatigue
- Fewer headaches, migraines ceased
- Decreased dental issues
- Weight stabilised
- Improvement in allergies

CHAPTER 15

Letting go

Hopes and aspirations

Melissa is a take-charge, conscientious young woman with a challenging professional career. Yet despite her success, it seemed that life was hard for Melissa; she appeared to carry all the worries of the world on her young shoulders. The anxiety that had plagued her since childhood just could not be controlled, even with medication and counselling. When Melissa enrolled in a breathing retraining course, it seemed to be a last desperate effort to end her constant struggle with 'anxiety attacks', as she called them.

Although she looked fit and athletic, Melissa's enrolment form ticked the boxes for shortness of breath, frequent deep breaths, tightness around the chest and excessive yawning. Melissa's initial breathing assessment using the capnometer showed reduced end-tidal carbon dioxide levels and indicated moderate over-breathing.

Melissa was charming and hard-working but seemed downcast during the first few days of the breathing retraining course. It appeared that she took control of her breathing retraining program like she did everything else in life: she was a star student and very diligent in carrying out her breathing exercises and doing everything to the letter. Yet much to her disappointment, her progress was slow and she began to berate herself for not achieving quicker results.

I reminded Melissa that she had been having these problems since childhood, and improving her breathing pattern would take time. I reassured her and explained that she just needed to do the breathing exercises and in time she would get results. I also explained to Melissa (as I explain to all of my clients) that however much she wanted to, she couldn't take control of her anxiety attacks and just get rid of them; she needed to give it time and let it go, otherwise the anxiety would continue to control her.

Melissa had a very busy schedule and it was months before she returned for a follow-up appointment. This time she looked like a different person – relaxed, glowing with good health and with a sparkle in her eyes! Her symptoms seemed to have vanished. When we did her breathing assessment, her carbon dioxide levels were not only in the normal range, they were at the optimal level. Melissa had not only done the breathing retraining homework, she had also learnt how to let go.

Since I started teaching breathing retraining in 1999, I have found that clients with anxiety and panic symptoms are often the most hard-working and conscientious people. Many of them, like Melissa, have very high expectations of themselves in everything they do, and some are perfectionists. I am in awe sometimes at how they can continue to work and live day by day with such debilitating symptoms. However, for these clients the disappointment and despondency they sometimes feel because they have not been able to control their anxiety and panic symptoms – despite time, effort, many different approaches and financial outlay – may be overwhelming.

In my classes I ask all clients to go easy on themselves, to give themselves a break and a pat on the back for small victories. Most of all, I ask them to be patient and give it time. I remind them that it is not their fault they have developed these symptoms. They are not weak – no-one would wish this upon themselves! And I remind them that despite the fact that they would happily take this condition by the throat and squeeze it to extinction, that's not going to happen – they have to learn to let it go. There is usually a wry smile at this point, as I think that is exactly what most of my clients would like to do with their anxiety and panic symptoms!

You are a survivor

If you are experiencing stress, anxiety or panic symptoms, remind yourself that you are a survivor, following in the footsteps of your ancestors, who managed to survive, generation after generation, often in dangerous or extreme conditions, precisely because of a well-honed and acute sense of danger and anxiety, combined with a heightened sense of self-preservation.

From my experience with clients, the key to successful breathing retraining lies in taking it slowly, doing the exercises and letting go, not in stressing out and trying to control the condition. As a bit of a confirmed control freak myself, I realise that this is never easy. However, we have to remind ourselves that there is never absolute control in life; we are fooling ourselves if we think there is.

'Relax and take deep breaths' is a common piece of well-meaning advice seen in self-help books on anxiety and panic attacks, and is sometimes the advice given by health professionals. Actually, the 'relax' part is fine, if you can do this (not easy if you are in the throes of a panic attack, or if you are really stressed out) but the deep-breathing advice is a big no-no and it's something you need to avoid if you are over-breathing.

In addition, it's best to avoid any activity, sport or exercise that emphasises or recommends deep breathing. For example, some forms of yoga, meditation or relaxation or some other forms of breathing exercises may require you to breathe more deeply or to mouth-breathe. If you are already over-breathing, why would you risk worsening your condition by taking deeper breaths? If you follow this piece of advice, increasing your breathing pattern may lead to an exacerbation of your symptoms. Figure 15.1 depicts the effect of taking bigger breaths if you are already over-breathing.

Exercise and sports sometimes have to be temporarily shelved when people are habitually over-breathing as they may be too difficult, due to shortness of breath or tightness in the chest. If you enjoy exercise and sporting activities, that's great, and in Part 2 of this book you will find some recommendations to help you pursue these activities without encouraging increases in your breathing pattern.

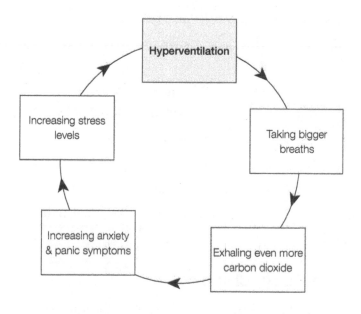

**Figure 15.1: The effects of taking bigger breaths
if you are already over-breathing**

Dare to hope

Sometimes when people have experienced stress, anxiety or panic attacks for a long time, they begin to lose hope of ever regaining control over their lives. Most of my clients have been to numerous doctors, specialists and therapists. Many have tried several other modalities, both complementary and alternative. These have all taken a toll in terms of expense, time and energy, and also in terms of maintaining a positive outlook. Sadly, some people experiencing anxiety and panic symptoms may begin to lose hope that they will ever be well again. 'You are my last hope,' many of my clients say. So sad, when a breathing retraining practitioner using an effective method should have been one of the first people they consulted – if only they had known which road to take.

If you or one of your loved ones is experiencing some of the issues discussed in this book, then there is a likelihood that these may be related to chronic or intermittent over-breathing. I would advise that you consult your doctor and then consider breathing retraining. Rest assured that the body is a finely tuned instrument and will do its utmost to protect itself, but you may need to provide some help by retraining your breathing to normal levels. The good news is that over-breathing – whether chronic or intermittent – is a habit and, like other habits, it can be changed.

The ultimate machine

Professor Buteyko referred to the body as the ultimate or 'the most complex machine'.[1] It has sophisticated renewal and regeneration powers that occur without us ever having to think about them, many of which I believe are yet to be discovered. When given a chance, the body's tendency is always to heal itself. With breathing retraining, we provide the best conditions for the body to do this, and that is something I have observed repeatedly since I started teaching.

During the early years, I must confess that at times I too was a little sceptical when my clients had complex health issues or severe, chronic symptoms. There were even a few times when I doubted that the method would be effective and thought, *This is too severe, I'm not sure this is going to work*, only to be proven wrong and to find, to my surprise, that it worked perfectly!

I am always struck by how much better people look even after the first few days of breathing retraining. And course participants often remark on how well their classmates look. They may even comment that some people look younger! After only a few days of improved breathing, clients seem to lose that tired grey pallor and they do sometimes look ten years younger, as if the weight of the world has been lifted off their shoulders.

'Life-changing' is a term that is often bandied about and is sometimes used in connection with superficial things. But when my clients say that they found the breathing retraining course life-changing, I know that their health and their quality of life have been profoundly improved. Best of all, they seem to have an increased vibrancy about them and a sparkle in their eyes, which was lacking prior to their breathing retraining course. Their zest for life has returned!

There is an old Chinese proverb that says, 'When the student is ready, the teacher appears.'

Are you ready? You too can learn to let go of your symptoms and achieve better health by following the breathing retraining strategies and techniques in Part 2 of this book.

Retrain your breathing pattern

A four-week program to improve your breathing

CHAPTER 16

Breathing and awareness

You can't change what you don't know

Before you start

Polepole (pronounced 'polly-polly') is Swahili for slow, or slow down. How do I know that *polepole* means 'slow down' in Swahili? And how is it relevant to breathing retraining? In my salad days (my early twenties) I, along with a group of five or six male climbers, managed to climb the highest mountain in Africa, Mount Kilimanjaro. Mount Kilimanjaro is beautiful, rising 5895 metres way above the clouds between Kenya and Tanzania, and exudes an air of awe and majesty. Even though it is not far from the equator, it is freezing cold towards its summit and at certain times of the year, snow and ice can be seen there. Believe me, this was not a walk in the park. And afterwards, those who knew me had a great laugh, as I have never been known for my sporting prowess or love of physical activity. An eight-hour shift as a nurse or a bit of dancing were as active as I got.

It took us three days to reach the summit. Just about everyone who climbed Kilimanjaro, with the exception of our guides, developed altitude sickness, including nausea, vomiting and splitting headaches, as well as aching muscles from climbing. With the benefit of hindsight, I now realise that for someone like myself, who had never been sporty or athletic, and whose only preparation was a walk along the beach at Malindi in Kenya, this was a major achievement. On the way up we kept meeting very fit, experienced, mostly male, Alpine climbers on their way down who had failed to reach the top. Why? Precisely because they were so fit and eager – they went up too quickly and had not taken the time to acclimatise to the reduced air pressure. In our group, our Kenyan guides kept saying, '*Polepole, polepole,*' and did not allow anyone to climb too quickly. So unlike those very fit, experienced – but in this case, unsuccessful – climbers, we took the climb at a slow, careful pace and, as a result, we all made it to the top!

The important point is that the body needs
time to gradually acclimatise to change.

Admittedly, acclimatising to the reduced air pressures on Mount Kilimanjaro is a different process from slowly raising carbon dioxide levels in the body for someone who is over-breathing. But the principle of *polepole* is exactly the same: the body needs time to gradually acclimatise to change.

Don't worry, I am not going to suggest that you climb a mountain or even undertake a fitness regimen or a strenuous exercise program. In fact, I recommend that you avoid strenuous exercise at the start of this program until your breathing pattern has improved and you can comfortably nose-breathe. I also advise that you take it slowly and master each stage before attempting the next.

I highly recommend that you take the time to read the earlier chapters in this book before you start your breathing retraining program, so that you can understand the processes involved in improving your breathing pattern and the way that breathing is linked to stress, anxiety and panic symptoms.

Before we get started, there are a few things to remember. It is important to take the following program week by week as set out, in order to achieve the best results. Don't be tempted to sprint ahead like those fit, eager and experienced climbers on Mount Kilimanjaro. What you are going to achieve in the next four weeks (or longer, if you need more time) is a gradual acclimatisation to a higher and *normalised* level of carbon dioxide and consequently reduced anxiety and panic symptoms, and better sleep. So *polepole* and take your time!

As mentioned previously, research has suggested that some people with anxiety and panic symptoms are sensitive to increases in carbon dioxide, even increases within the normal range.[1, 2] These increases in carbon dioxide may cause symptoms to worsen and may make some people feel uncomfortable or provoke anxiety and panic attacks. Therefore, it is necessary to proceed slowly at first until you acclimatise and this sensitivity is reduced. For this reason, the breathing retraining strategies are introduced gradually. Everyone is different, so if you find you are struggling with a particular week, and need more time, feel free to repeat that week before proceeding. Don't be tempted to rush ahead; speed is not important. What *is* important is improving your breathing pattern and your health.

For some people the adjustment could take six or more weeks, depending on how diligent they are and on their individual response to the breathing retraining exercises. For someone with severe over-breathing or who has had anxiety since childhood, one would not expect significant changes within a week! However, I have found from my practice that most people will *begin* to feel better within days. Patience is a virtue, they say.

Getting started

Depending on your schedule, you will need to do an awareness day or, even better, a couple of awareness days, before starting the breathing retraining exercises in the next chapter. I recommend that you acquire a folder for your homework, so that you can keep records and monitor your response and your progress. You will find it easier to stay on track that way.

For your binder or folder you will need to:

- Make two copies of the breathing questionnaire (see Table 5.1 on page 62) – one for your initial baseline assessment and one for the end of your four-week program.
- Make four copies of the daily diary page in this chapter (Table 16.1 on page 193) – one for each of the next four weeks.

Before you start, complete the breathing questionnaire from Chapter 5 (Table 5.1) to give you a baseline breathing assessment.

Check your results on the pages following the questionnaire to see how your assessment went.

Develop breathing awareness

Over-breathing is essentially a habit. When people ask what I do, I usually say, 'I teach people how to breathe.' Then they laugh and look at me with astonishment. Surely everyone knows how to breathe or they wouldn't be alive? I then qualify this, and say, 'I teach people how to improve their breathing.'

Over-breathing is essentially a habit. The first step to changing any habit is awareness – you can't change what you don't know!

Conventional wisdom says that you can't change what you don't know, and this is very true when it comes to changing and improving your breathing pattern. The first step to changing any habit is awareness. So for the awareness day/s and in the weeks ahead, I would like you to observe your breathing pattern so that you become aware of what you need to improve. You may, of course, also consult loved ones or trusted friends for feedback on your breathing. They may be more aware of your breathing pattern than you think – they may even have noticed things about your breathing pattern that you were not aware of.

I recommend that you begin your awareness day/s on an average day of the week, with an average amount of stress, so that you can get a good indication of your breathing pattern.

If you choose a weekend or a day when you feel relaxed and rested, you may not gain the same insight.

On these days just observe your breathing pattern, your posture and your symptoms from time to time as you go about your daily activities – working, moving, walking, exercising, eating and speaking. Notice how your breathing pattern relates to your symptoms. If you find that you are mouth-breathing, shallow-breathing, sighing or yawning excessively at any time, make a mental or written note. Through your observations you will become aware of the things you need to focus on and improve during your breathing retraining program.

Conventional wisdom also says that it takes three weeks to change a habit. A disordered breathing pattern is an acquired habit and changing it is like any other habit: you substitute a different habit, in this case an improved breathing pattern.

However, as breathing is very instinctual, for some people it may take longer than three weeks to change their breathing pattern, although they will begin to feel improvement within a week or two, sometimes even within the first few days.

Your symptoms may be greatly improved or even eliminated after a couple of weeks, but I recommend that you continue with the full program for a minimum of four weeks. This will allow you to become more confident with your breathing pattern and avoid reverting to over-breathing in times of increased stress. For most people I find it generally takes around four to six weeks for the improved breathing pattern to become automatic.

During the four weeks of your breathing retraining program, I recommend that you complete your diary page (Table 16.1) every day – preferably every evening before bed – in order to monitor your progress.

	Date	Date	Date	Date	Date	Date	Date
TABLE 16.1: DAILY DIARY PAGE Make four copies of this diary page, one for each week. **Each evening before bed, please tick your answers and insert a sleep score as applicable below.**							
My nose was blocked at times							
My chest felt tight at times							
I was short of breath at times							
I sighed or yawned a lot							
I could hear my breathing at times							
I was mostly nose-breathing							
I was mostly mouth-breathing							
I was shallow-breathing at times							
Most of the time my breathing felt okay							
I felt anxious at times							
I felt stressed at times							
I had a headache							
I felt really tired all day							
My muscles ached							
I felt spaced out							
I had palpitations							
I felt dizzy at times							
I had a panic attack/s							
If you had anxiety or panic attacks today, please describe your breathing at the time:							
I was short of breath							
I was breathing faster							
I was mouth-breathing							
My posture was poor							
I did not notice my breathing or posture							
Sleep – last night:							
I had difficulty getting to sleep							
I woke up during the night							
I couldn't get back to sleep							
I snored (according to partner)							
I woke with a dry mouth							
I slept mainly on my side							
I slept mainly on my front							
I slept mainly on my back							
Overall sleep score out of 10 (10/10 = excellent)	/10	/10	/10	/10	/10	/10	/10
I am avoiding situations to prevent symptoms. (Please circle answer. Ignore if not applicable)	Yes No Unsure	Yes No Unsure	Yes No Unsure	Yes No Unsure	Yes No Unsure	Yes No Unsure	Yes No Unsure

Remember:

- Monitor your breathing and posture during your awareness
  day/s as suggested, in order to:
  - gain an awareness of how you breathe,
  - find out how your symptoms are related to your breathing,
    and
  - discover what you need to improve.
- Record your observations on your daily diary page (Table
  16.1) before bed.
- Continue to be aware of your breathing pattern during the
  next few weeks of your program.

Constant mouth-breathing almost invariably
means that you are over-breathing.

You may need to ask a partner, family member or a trusted
friend for feedback on some of these questions contained in the
breathing questionnaire and your daily diary page, e.g. posture,
snoring or nose-breathing, if you are unsure. Breathing is so
automatic that we generally don't notice how we breathe on
a daily basis. You may have been over-breathing for months
or even years and therefore it may have become automatic to
over-breathe, particularly in times of stress. Some people are
convinced that they nose-breathe all the time and are quite taken
aback when I gently point out that they are mouth-breathing.
So, enlisting help may be necessary to be able to answer some
of these questions. You could try recording your breathing at

night if you wish, but this is not really necessary. You will know if you wake yourself up with snoring, or if you wake up with a dry mouth or a headache, or if you wake anxious and panicky. When this happens there is a significant chance that you have been mouth-breathing while sleeping.

On the other hand, some people may be acutely aware that something is not right with their breathing. In fact, I have found that some of my clients are so out of touch with a normal breathing pattern that when I ask them to take a normal breath in, they say they don't know what normal means any more. Don't be concerned if this applies to you also; just by becoming aware of your breathing pattern and by doing the exercises as suggested, your breathing will improve.

You will begin to notice *how* you breathe, whether you predominantly mouth-breathe or nose-breathe, whether your breathing is loud or soft, whether you sigh or yawn excessively and so on. You may begin to notice a link between your breathing pattern and your symptoms, which will become extremely helpful when it comes to controlling and eventually eliminating the stress, anxiety and panic symptoms.

Then, with the knowledge gained from this awareness exercise, you will be able to move on and start the four-week program. Each week I will suggest some practical strategies you can adopt, which will help you improve your breathing pattern step by step.

Posture matters

You will also need to become familiar with your posture, as good posture is essential for effective and efficient breathing and for correct use of the diaphragm. When we are slumped or stooped, the diaphragm cannot perform to its potential and breathing becomes more difficult. In addition, most of the tiny air sacs (the alveoli) in the lungs where gas exchange takes place are located further down in the lungs, and fewer air sacs are available at the top of the lungs. The bottom line is that poor posture will compress the diaphragm and other breathing muscles and make breathing more difficult.

Adopting a C-shaped posture does not allow for effective air exchange. Without altering your posture, try right now to get an idea of what it is like. Score your posture (even better, get someone else to score your posture when you are unaware) in Table 16.2.

Posture scores are based on the following:

- C shape/leaning or slouching forwards
- bending in the middle/back curved
- shoulders slumping forwards or shoulders up towards ears
- tension in shoulder, neck or jaw.

TABLE 16.2: POSTURE CHECK	
	Your score
Back straight	/5
Shoulders back, relaxed and down	/3
Neck and jaw relaxed	/1
Chin slightly up	/1
Total (Excellent posture = 10/10)	/10

How did you go? From my practice, I have found that many people who are stressed or who experience anxiety and panic symptoms have poor posture. Their shoulders are sometimes raised and thrust forwards. Their back is curved into a C shape and their body is slumped forwards. Due to a combination of poor posture, stress and anxiety, they may have tension in the neck and shoulders or in the jaw. This may lead to the development of tension headaches, particularly if the position is held in front of a desk or a computer over time.

When we are anxious, our posture generally deteriorates. Fortunately, posture is something we can improve over time just by becoming more aware of it and by reminding ourselves to adopt an upright posture during the day, particularly when we feel stressed or anxious.

Monitoring your progress

Sometimes my clients are genuinely very surprised when they attend a follow-up review after three weeks and I ask them to tick which symptoms on their enrolment sheet have improved or have been eliminated since their enrolment. 'Did I tick that?' they ask in amazement, completely forgetting what their symptoms were before they started the course!

Obtaining a baseline assessment of your breathing pattern and posture will enable you to monitor your progress during the next few weeks. Sometimes improvements are gradual rather than noticeable from day to day, so monitoring your progress in your daily diary each evening and repeating the breathing questionnaire (Chapter 5, Table 5.1) at the end of four weeks will help you to see improvements more readily and to stay motivated and on track while completing your objectives.

In the following chapters I have summarised the breathing retraining strategies and activities at the end of each week to remind you what you need to do. Don't forget to complete your daily diary page every evening before bed.

AWARENESS DAY/S CHECKLIST	
ACTIVITIES	❏ Complete the **breathing questionnaire** (Chapter 5, Table 5.1) **before** you start awareness day/s. ❏ Complete the **daily diary** page (Chapter 16, Table 16.1) each day before bed.
BREATHING	❏ During the day, become aware of your **breathing pattern**. When moving, walking, speaking or exercising, and particularly while under stress, notice your breathing pattern. Are you mouth-breathing, sighing, yawning, shallow breathing, breathing faster or breathing loudly? Record your observations in your diary this evening.
POSTURE	❏ While engaged in your daily living activities, become aware of your **posture** and make a mental note of what you need to improve.
SYMPTOMS	❏ Notice any stress, anxiety and panic **symptoms**. When do they happen? What makes them worse? Notice your breathing while you are stressed, anxious or having a panic attack. Is it more audible, or shallower, or faster? Are you avoiding certain places or situations? Record your observations in your diary each evening.
SLEEP	❏ How did you **sleep** last night? Are you having difficulty getting to sleep or staying asleep? Are you waking up snoring or in a panic? How many times did you wake last night? Record these in your diary.

CHAPTER 17

Week 1: Healthy breathing habits

Breathing should be appropriate for the activity

Aims and objectives:

- Discover the three pillars for healthy breathing.
- Discover the Nose-breathing Pyramid.
- Learn how to unblock your nose.
- Learn how to reduce anxiety and panic symptoms.

If you have completed the breathing questionnaire and the awareness day/s strategies described in the previous chapter, you are now ready to start your breathing retraining program.

Three pillars for healthy breathing

This is the exciting part! Following your breathing awareness day/s, you will be keen to make a start on improving your breathing pattern and reducing symptoms. By now you are becoming more familiar with your breathing pattern from your initial observations and from monitoring your breathing and your symptoms. You will need to continue to be aware of your breathing and your posture for the next few weeks.

Today, at the start of your program, you will start to implement some strategies to improve your breathing pattern and manage and reduce stress, anxiety and panic attacks. We will start with the Three Pillars for Healthy Breathing set out in Table 17.1 and then move on to the Nose-breathing Pyramid.

TABLE 17.1: THREE PILLARS FOR HEALTHY BREATHING		
Pillar 1	Pillar 2	Pillar 3
Nose-breathe only	Always breathe gently	Adopt correct posture

Pillar 1: Nose-breathe only

It is important to begin to normalise the volume of air breathed in and out, and this is achieved primarily through nose-breathing. So, from today onwards, make sure to check your breathing from time to time and ensure that you are always nose-breathing. Remember, you need to nose-breathe both in and out.

In particular, observe how you breathe as you move about, sit down or get up. Do you exhale with a deep sigh through your mouth as you sit down? This is an indication that you may be over-breathing. Are you continuously nose-breathing as you walk around? Is your mouth open in concentration as you watch TV or focus on your work or study or sit in front of the computer? It may be helpful to explain to your family or a trusted friend or colleague that you are doing a breathing retraining program and ask them to remind you to close your mouth if they catch you mouth-breathing.

By 'close your mouth' I don't mean that you need to clench your teeth together. Gently close your lips, so that your tongue is located just behind your upper teeth. Clenching your teeth may lead to tension and an aching jaw.

SEVERE ANXIETY OR PANIC SYMPTOMS?

If your symptoms are severe, e.g. daily panic attacks or waking at night with panic attacks, nose-breathing may make you feel a little anxious or uncomfortable initially. If that is the case, then you may need to practise gentle nose-breathing for five or ten minutes a few times each day until nose-breathing becomes more comfortable, then continue with the program.

Remember, nose-breathing is the cornerstone of healthy breathing and is key to developing better breathing habits and improving your breathing pattern. So I strongly recommend that you keep your mouth closed, except of course when you are eating, drinking or speaking. When we mouth-breathe, not only are we over-breathing and increasing the volume of air inhaled, we also bypass some important protective mechanisms. Evolution has meant that our noses are designed specifically to make sure that the air we inhale is just right for our air-tubes and lungs, as can be seen from Table 17.2 overleaf. The bottom line is: mouth-breathing is not a healthy habit!

For some people in the initial stages of breathing retraining, nose-breathing may feel a little uncomfortable. If this occurs, try to nose-breathe as much as you can; it will become easier with practice. If nose-breathing makes you feel anxious or panicky initially, this is not unusual. Remind yourself that you need to breathe gently through your nose, knowing that you are safe, that we are meant to nose-breathe, and that you are improving your breathing pattern. After a couple of days you will begin to feel more comfortable, and within a week most people are automatically breathing through the nose.

TABLE 17.2: NOSE-BREATHING VS MOUTH-BREATHING	
Nose-breathing	Mouth-breathing
The volume of air we inhale is reduced towards normal.	The volume of air is increased as there is more capacity.
The air we breathe in is: • slowed down and warmed in the nasal passages • humidified (picks up moisture from the nasal passages) • filtered (due to the cilia or little projections in the nose).	The air goes straight down, with no chance for: • warming • moistening or humidifying • filtration. While mouth-breathing we may be inhaling as much as four or five times the normal amount of air, as well as four or five times the amount of toxins and allergens, fumes, pollutants, smoke, moulds, pollens, dust mites, pet dander, etc.
As a general rule, due to a normal volume of air inhaled while nose-breathing, we retain sufficient carbon dioxide as we exhale – if we are gently nose-breathing in and out.	Constant mouth-breathing leads to an increased volume of air inhaled and exhaled, leading to over-breathing, excessive loss of carbon dioxide when exhaling, and symptoms such as anxiety and panic attacks.
We utilise the body's defence mechanisms located in the nose (the immune system) to ward off viruses and infections.	The body's natural defence mechanisms in the nose are bypassed, leading to colds, flu and increased allergies.

Pillar 2: Always breathe gently

Most of the time, your breathing should not be audible to you or anyone else, particularly while sitting or at rest. In previous chapters I hope I managed to dispel the modern myth that deep breathing is good for us. Breathing should be appropriate for the activity. In other words, when very active or playing strenuous sports, it's normal to breathe more deeply or audibly, but while sitting, standing or just walking around, you should not be able to hear yourself breathe.

While you are sitting at a desk or watching TV, or even walking at a normal pace, check that your breathing is *gentle*, in and out through the nose, and is not audible. Even while strolling around you should not be able to hear yourself breathe.

In the future, when you have mastered the first levels on the Nose-breathing Pyramid (on the next page), and if you want to do level 4 upwards (climbing stairs, running or exercising vigorously), it's okay to breathe a bit more audibly – but predominantly through the nose.

Pillar 3: Adopt correct posture

When I assess my clients' breathing patterns using capnometry, I am surprised how often improving posture leads to an immediate improvement in breathing pattern – including an improvement in end-tidal carbon dioxide levels. There are several flow-on benefits from improved posture. Recent studies suggest that adopting good posture can improve the stress response and also improve mood and memory, as well as boost self-esteem.[1]

The bottom line is: be aware of your posture during your breathing retraining program. Always stand tall: back straight and shoulders back, down and relaxed. Good posture is essential for good breathing. From the breathing questionnaire, and from monitoring your posture, you will probably have started to realise its importance. Good posture is not only aimed at looking good, it is very important for effective breathing and for correct use of the diaphragm and chest muscles. Therefore, improved posture equals improved breathing.

There are some extra bonuses if you stand tall. Correct posture will lead to:

- correct use of the diaphragm
- correct use of the intercostal (breathing) muscles
- less tension in neck, shoulders and ribcage, and, therefore, fewer headaches
- ability to use the lower air sacs more effectively, therefore improving exchange of gases in the lungs
- and, of course, looking and feeling more confident and in control.

So this week, whether you are walking, sitting at the computer, standing or relaxing, please continue to focus on your posture from time to time and adopt the recommendations to improve your posture. When you sit in a chair, ensure that your buttocks are right up against the back of the chair, not halfway across the seat. This will help to prevent you from slumping forwards and adopting a C-shaped posture.

The Nose-breathing Pyramid

Depending on your fitness level and your ability, this graduated program will help you to acclimatise to nose-breathing comfortably and effortlessly during the next few weeks. Begin with gentle nose-breathing while seated, then when you are comfortable with that you can progress to nose-breathing while walking. Later on you will progress to walking up an incline and taking the stairs while nose-breathing. This hypothetical pyramid in Figure 17.1 includes being able to comfortably nose-breathe as shown, starting with nose-breathing while seated, then moving on to more strenuous activities as you progress during the next few weeks.

| 8. Exercising/playing sports |
| 7. Running |
| 6. Short bursts of jogging |
| 5. Climbing steps or stairs |
| 4. Walking up an incline |
| 3. Walking faster |
| 2. Strolling/walking |
| 1. While seated |

Figure 17.1: The Nose-breathing Pyramid
Options 1 to 5 are recommended targets to aim for in
the next few weeks. Options 6 to 8 are optional.

As mentioned in Chapter 9, we increase carbon dioxide levels when we move or exercise, as energy requirements are increased. In fact, the more energetic we are, the more carbon dioxide we produce, but we need to learn to retain carbon dioxide by breathing appropriately for the activity, and this includes gentle nose-breathing while seated or walking. Eventually, with practice, you will be able to predominantly nose-breathe during more strenuous activities such as jogging, running or sports without feeling the need to gulp air or feeling breathless. (For those keen on exercise, the good news is that nose-breathing will help with endurance, but right now we are focusing on the basics.)

CAUTION – take it slowly

As I am not with you in person to guide you, I recommend that you start with baby steps and then progress slowly. Sports and strenuous exercise are optional. However, if you would like to get fit or take up a sport (or if you currently do sports or vigorous exercise), you will need to avoid strenuous exercise in the short term until you can comfortably nose-breathe at each level, starting at the bottom of the pyramid. Always get a medical check-up before starting any exercise program.

By nose-breathing gently you will reduce the volume of air breathed in and out. This will ensure that you begin to retain carbon dioxide and normalise your levels of this essential gas.

It will take time to adapt to the increasing levels of carbon dioxide that are a natural part of increasing exercise. This is even more important for people experiencing anxiety and panic disorders, where some may be sensitive to slight – though normal – increases in carbon dioxide. The nose-breathing levels on the pyramid provide a graduated approach you can take at your own pace over the four-week program to help you acclimatise to increasing levels of carbon dioxide to a normal range. Once you are comfortably able to nose-breathe constantly at one level on the pyramid, you may progress to the next level. This week we will start nose-breathing at level 1 on the pyramid and, during the week, progress to level 2.

> It's very important to let your breathing dictate your pace and slow down or stop if you can't nose-breathe.

So, starting today, whether you are sitting or strolling around, begin to observe your breathing pattern and try to ensure that you are nose-breathing gently at all times, both when inhaling and while exhaling.

How to unblock your nose

Initially, some people struggle with a blocked nose. If this happens to you and your nose keeps blocking, I recommend that you use this short breathing pause to unblock your nose:

- Sit or stand.
- Take a normal breath *in* and *out* through your nose. If your nose is totally blocked, sneak a small breath in through your mouth.
- Pinch your nose after the out breath and then, keeping your mouth closed, slowly count five seconds in your mind. It may help to say, 'One thousand, two thousand, three thousand, four thousand, five thousand,' slowly in your

mind (not out loud). This is equivalent to five seconds. Or you can use the stopwatch on your mobile phone.

- Let go of your nose, then breathe in again through your nose, *but be sure to keep your mouth closed*. Do not allow yourself to mouth-breathe after this pause, even if you feel like breathing through your mouth. Continue to breathe through your nose. You may find that your nasal passages will crackle as mucus is shifted. If this happens, just blow your nose and continue to nose-breathe gently.

Do not hold your breath for longer than five seconds. You may need to do this exercise now and then for a day or two as you adjust to nose-breathing. Persevere with nose-breathing and always blow your nose and try to keep it clear. Try to unblock your nose before it is totally blocked, to avoid the mouth-breathing habit. It may take a few days before the blocking stops entirely but it does get easier, the more you continue to nose-breathe.

Avoid overuse of this exercise as it may cause a headache in some people – just use it occasionally to unblock your nose.

Avoid medicated over-the-counter nasal sprays to unblock your nose, as these often have a rebound effect. As soon as you stop using them, your nose quickly reverts to blocking up again. These sprays may work initially but they can affect the delicate mucous membranes in the nose and lead to increased blocking if used for prolonged periods.

If you are struggling, a steam inhalation may help. Avoid using oils such as eucalyptus in steam inhalations as they may be a little harsh and can irritate the mucous membranes in the nasal passages. You might also like to try a nasal spray that has normal saline (salt) in sterile water for a day or two, if nose-blocking remains a problem. These are fairly inexpensive and are available at pharmacies. However, just unblocking your nose and giving yourself time to adapt may be the best remedy.

Dealing with anxiety and panic symptoms

During stress, anxiety or a panic attack, the body goes into a state similar to the fight-or-flight response and is, therefore, focusing on survival. At the beginning of a panic attack, everything may seem to happen in seconds, and your focus may be on several different things, such as trying to appear normal, wanting to escape, fear of passing out, fear of embarrassment, and even fear of dying. Stress hormones dominate the body during an anxiety or panic attack and the fight-or-flight response is heightened and activated.

Practise these exercises when you are not so stressed or anxious so that you will know what to do in the event that you start to feel anxious or panicky.

Act like a caveman

Imagine that a caveman senses danger. Let's say he glimpses a predator, such as a wild animal, lurking behind a rock. What would he do? We can safely assume that he would go into the fight-or-flight mode. But the last thing he would want to do is make his presence obvious by breathing heavily! Therefore, it stands to reason he will initially try to avoid deep breathing or noisy breathing. If he decides to run and make an escape, once he is out of earshot he may then begin breathing more deeply in order to make it to safety.

At the start of a panic attack your attention may not be focused on breathing at all, but quite naturally on fleeing or escaping. However, it is generally over-breathing or hyperventilation that induces and sustains panic attacks; therefore, your focus needs to be on your breathing pattern and on controlling and reducing over-breathing.

But how do I do that, you may ask. I advise my clients experiencing stress, anxiety and panic symptoms that they initiate the Controlled Breathing Exercise as described on the next page at the first sign of symptoms. Practise the Controlled Breathing Exercise so that you feel more confident when you begin to experience anxiety or panic.

Adopt the horse-riding position

Some of my clients have found this position very helpful to control symptoms when practising the Controlled Breating Exercise.

- Sit right at the edge of a kitchen chair, office chair or dining chair with your weight balanced between your bottom and your feet.
- Place your feet about hip-width apart.
- Keep your back straight and your shoulders back, relaxed and down as if you are on a horse.
- Keep your head up as if you are looking into the distance to see where you are going.
- Do the Controlled Breathing Exercise.

The Controlled Breathing Exercise

My clients have found that the Controlled Breathing Exercise (Figure 17.2) is a very effective way to prevent or ward off anxiety and panic symptoms. Initially it may take a minute or two for the anxiety and panic symptoms to subside. I have found that as clients become more confident with this routine and their breathing improves, they can stop a panic attack in its tracks with a few breaths. With practice, you can become more confident and proficient at controlling and overcoming symptoms while carrying out the Controlled Breathing Exercise.

FIGURE 17.2: CONTROLLED BREATHING EXERCISE TO PREVENT AND CONTROL SYMPTOMS

You can sit or stand for this breathing exercise.

    At the first sign of anxiety or panic symptoms:

- Adopt the horse-riding position if possible.
- Close your mouth so that your tongue rests comfortably, gently touching the back of your upper front teeth.
- Focus on your breathing.
- Nose-breathe *slowly* and *gently* – you should not be able to hear yourself breathe.
- Initiate a *slow, gentle* nose-breathing routine as you say in your mind, 'Breathe in – 2 – 3 – 4, breathe out – 2 – 3 – 4.'
- Check your posture: your back should be straight and shoulders back, down and relaxed.
- Release any tension in your jaw, neck and shoulders.
- Avoid counting breaths per minute.
- Do not be frightened to breathe; reassure yourself that your body is taking care of itself.
- Continue the exercise for a minute or two.

To calm down your breathing and avert or alleviate symptoms, take time out and focus on the Controlled Breathing Exercise.

Like my client Jo in the story in Chapter 5, you will find it helpful to:

- recognise when your breathing is off
- take time out
- take action (such as controlled breathing) to prevent the attacks from happening.

As your breathing improves through implementing the range of strategies recommended during these four weeks, the symptoms and panic attacks will become less frequent and will eventually cease. The good news is that you can do the Controlled Breathing Exercise anywhere, and no-one is aware that you are doing it.

An alternative to the Controlled Breathing Exercise that some people find helpful is to walk or move around for a few minutes while *gently* nose-breathing. This will help to simulate the flight part of the fight-or-flight response and hopefully get rid of some of the excess adrenaline that is produced during an anxiety or panic attack. In addition, the extra carbon dioxide produced by moving around – and which will be retained by gentle nose-breathing – will help to reduce the panic symptoms.

Avoid counting the number of breaths per minute in an effort to keep your breathing within the normal range, as this may increase your anxiety and stress levels. The Controlled Breathing Exercise (depending on the rate of your inner counting) will usually mean that you are breathing at a rate of around 8–10 breaths per minute, which is nicely within the optimal rate of 8–14 breaths per minute.

If you shallow-breathe

If you find that you are shallow-breathing at any time, or developing a hunger for air, I would recommend that you do the Controlled Breathing Exercise, as explained above. Shallow-breathing is a form of disordered breathing and it may be followed by a period of sighing, yawning and over-breathing, leading to anxiety or panic attacks, so it's important to change to a more efficient way of breathing as soon as possible.

Shallow-breathing may also mean that you have already filled your lungs by over-breathing so there is insufficient room left for a full breath. It may sound strange to hear that you need to slow down your breathing and breathe more gently when all you want to do is to take deeper breaths! It's paradoxical that improving posture, and slowing down and controlling your breathing, will help to dispel that air-hunger feeling. Do not be frightened to breathe, though; as long as you are gently nose-breathing while doing the Controlled Breathing Exercise you will be fine.

Take another look at Table 1.1 in Chapter 1, which contrasts normal breathing and over-breathing. The first guideline is that breathing should be effortless. Your breathing may not feel effortless right now, but it will begin to improve within a short time.

Relaxation and deep breathing are out ... slow, controlled breathing is in

Very commonly, people experiencing anxiety and panic attacks are advised by well-meaning friends, websites or even some health professionals to 'relax and take deep breaths', or to breathe deeply from the diaphragm. In my opinion this may not be appropriate advice, given that people experiencing anxiety and panic symptoms are already over-breathing. Why would you need to take deep breaths if you are already over-breathing or hyperventilating? It just doesn't make sense.

Trying to relax while in the grip of an anxiety or panic attack is a bit like trying to stop the tide.

Deep breathing is not recommended because:

- You are most likely already taking deeper breaths while you are anxious or about to experience a panic attack. Deepening breathing is part of the stress response, so why would you want to breathe more deeply and prolong or worsen the attack? Therefore what is needed is slow, controlled (not deep) breathing.
- As you are most likely already acutely aware, trying to relax is very difficult while in the grip of an anxiety or panic attack – it's a bit like trying to stop the tide.

What some people may find helpful is *controlled* breathing from the diaphragm.

Belly/abdominal or diaphragmatic breathing

You may have been advised to breathe from the diaphragm. However, breathing from the diaphragm is not easy, unless you're already an expert on this and you can do it while calm. Also, while a couple of minutes of diaphragmatic breathing now and then may be okay, if it is done for prolonged periods, breathing from the diaphragm – or 'belly breathing' as some people call it – can lead to very sore abdominal muscles. (See Chapter 8 for more information on abdominal breathing.) It is possible to deep-breathe and to *over-breathe* from the diaphragm, which is not a good habit to adopt. If you find that a minute or two of belly breathing now and then helps, that's fine, but don't overdo it. We don't need to reinforce the deep-breathing habit.

For these reasons, I don't teach belly breathing. But I have found that when clients improve posture and learn to nose-breathe gently, they automatically start to breathe correctly from the diaphragm.

Sleep

Most people with high stress levels, anxiety and panic symptoms need to improve their sleep. For now, try to sleep *only* on your side – never on your back – which will help you improve your breathing pattern and your sleep. (If you have a medical condition or injury that precludes you from sleeping on your side, consult your doctor.) Place a cushion or a pillow behind your back to stop you from rolling while asleep.

WEEK 1: BREATHING RETRAINING CHECKLIST	
ACTIVITIES	❑ Continue to be aware of your breathing pattern. ❑ Adopt the three **pillars** for healthy breathing. ❑ Nose-breathe while doing levels 1 and 2 on the **pyramid**. If possible, avoid the other levels until later. ❑ Complete your **daily diary** page each evening.
BREATHING	❑ Learn the **nose-unblocking** exercise. ❑ Avoid mouth-breathing. ❑ **Nose-breathe** gently throughout the day. Whether sitting, standing, moving or walking, nose-breathe only. Let your breathing dictate your pace. Slow down or stop if you can't nose-breathe.
POSTURE	❑ Be aware of your posture throughout the day and try to maintain an upright but relaxed posture (pillar 3 for good breathing).
SYMPTOMS	❑ Learn the **Controlled Breathing Exercise** and the **horse-riding position**. At the first sign of symptoms, take time out and initiate this exercise as described.
SLEEP	❑ Sleep only on your side.

CHAPTER 18

Week 2: Breathing, sleep and mood

No cell is an island ... everything works in unison

Aims and objectives

- Learn how to improve your sleep.
- Discover strategies to help you relax and make your breathing more comfortable.
- Discover the best exercise to improve your breathing pattern, mood and sleep.
- Learn strategies to improve carbon dioxide levels.

Most people with anxiety and panic symptoms do not sleep well and they are constantly tired and stressed as a result. This week we will be looking in more detail at ways to improve your breathing pattern, your sense of wellbeing and your sleep.

You may have heard the saying 'No man is an island'. We could say the same thing about the body: 'No cell in the body is an island'. Everything about the body is interrelated and no system in the body works in isolation – your breathing pattern, your sleep, your immune system, your nutrition, and your lifestyle and exercise levels all work together in an integrated and holistic way in order to keep you healthy. Therefore, if one component is out of balance, other areas are also thrown out of kilter: stress leads to over-breathing and over-breathing leads to anxiety and panic symptoms. Habitual over-breathing can also lead to poor sleep, and consequently to fatigue, increasing stress levels and other symptoms.

The majority of my clients report that they do not sleep well. They may have difficulty getting to sleep, or they may wake up several times a night, or their sleep is not refreshing and they wake up in the morning feeling tired. This impacts on their overall health and vitality and increases their stress levels and their symptoms.

Improving your breathing pattern during the day will help you improve your breathing – and your sleep – at night. And, of course, this also works in reverse: improving your breathing pattern at night will lead to adequate refreshing sleep and, therefore, help to reduce daytime fatigue, improve your immune system, increase wellbeing and aid in withstanding stress during the day.

Sleep is a time of rest, regeneration and repair.
Without proper sleep we cannot perform well
or concentrate the next day, and we are more
likely to be stressed and anxious as a result.

The stress-anxiety-insomnia cycle

Do you keep a glass of water on your bedside table because you wake up with a dry mouth during the night or in the morning? Or do you find that you wake a few times during the night to visit the bathroom? Do you wake yourself snoring or do you sometimes wake in panic? Do you wake up in the morning with a headache?

These are signs that you are most likely mouth-breathing while asleep and are therefore over-breathing during the night. Your sleep is probably not as refreshing as it should be and you will most likely be feeling fatigued, stressed out, lacking in concentration or tired and achy the next day. Refreshing sleep is critical to reduce anxiety, improve health and wellbeing, and help the body to heal from the effects of stress.

These are the strategies I recommend you adopt to improve your breathing pattern and your sleep:

- Avoid eating a heavy meal within two hours (preferably three hours) of bedtime. By heavy, I mean a meal containing animal protein or with a high fat content.
- Also, avoid caffeine, alcohol, coffee and strong tea for at least four hours before bedtime.
- Initiate a bedtime routine: unwind with quiet time, play soft music or do some light reading.
- Dim the lights an hour before bed. In nature, the body produces melatonin, the sleep hormone, in response to fading light, starting at twilight. If we artificially keep the lights bright, we may not produce enough of this important

hormone and we may have trouble sleeping, or we may wake up in the middle of the night.

- Avoid using electronic equipment, such as TVs, mobile phones, tablets or laptops in the hour preceding bedtime as the light they emit may interfere with your melatonin levels. Blue light produced by electronic screens has the same effect as morning light and may have a similar effect to caffeine and keep us awake. There are apps available to filter blue light on mobile phones and tablets, but there is still some controversy surrounding these.

- *Always* sleep on your side; never sleep on your back. Why? Because when you are asleep on your back, chances are your jaw will drop open and you will start mouth-breathing. Mouth-breathing increases the volume of air you are inhaling and will lead to over-breathing, snoring, possible sinus issues and waking up with a dry mouth. Sleeping on your side will help to improve breathing, as your jaw is not so likely to drop open. (If you snore, this sleeping position will also help to improve your sleep – and also your partner's sleep.)

  - Place a cushion or a pillow behind your back for a few nights to ensure that you do not roll over.

  - If you have a partner, ask them to wake you if they find you on your back. Or, even better, they may feel inclined to help you to roll onto your side while you are not fully awake.

- Sleep with your mouth closed.

  - If your nose is blocked, unblock your nose using the instructions and strategies suggested in Week 1.

  - Ensure your nose is unblocked during the day to reinforce the nose-breathing habit. You will know that your night-time breathing pattern is improving when you start waking up feeling more refreshed, with more energy and ready to start the day.

Food, breathing and sleep

After eating a large meal, the body needs to increase energy levels and metabolism in order to digest that meal. Therefore, with this increased metabolism, the pulse rate and the breathing rate usually rise – this is normal and to be expected. However, if the person is already over-breathing and they eat a large meal close to bedtime, this can lead to increased symptoms and to trouble sleeping. It can take four hours or more for some food items, like meats, to be dealt with in the stomach before making their way into the small intestine.

I recommend not eating a large meal within two hours of bedtime (preferably three or four hours), depending on the meal. A large, fatty, protein-heavy meal can take more than four hours to digest. A snack is okay as it will be digested faster. For example, a piece of fruit on its own will clear the stomach in around twenty minutes. While asleep, the body needs to go into repair and regenerate mode. We do not cope well with digesting a large meal while sleeping, particularly if we are already over-breathing.

Some people do not tolerate dairy produce very well and this may contribute to poor sleep. Avoid dairy for a few days, especially before bedtime, to see if this helps.

Recent research suggests that a diet high in fibre, fruits and vegetables, and whole grains, and low in saturated fat, processed food and sugar improves sleep quality.[1] This study found that improved nutrition leads to improved quality in the deeper levels of sleep.

In addition to implementing these food recommendations, walking as described later in this chapter in 'Walk your way to better health and breathing' may also help you to improve your sleep pattern.

Do you wake up between 1 a.m. and 3 a.m.?

Constantly waking up between 1 a.m. and 3 a.m. may be due to various reasons, not least over-breathing. If you wake with a dry mouth, then you are most likely mouth-breathing and, therefore, over-breathing. Sleeping on your side will help; also see low blood sugar (hypoglycaemia) suggestions below.

Low blood sugar

Hypoglycaemia, or low blood sugar levels, may also be a factor contributing to poor sleep in some people. The remedy is to eat a light snack before bed: for example, hummus on wholemeal toast or a cracker, or a few nuts, or perhaps some avocado. As animal protein is harder to digest, make sure to get adequate protein during the day, rather than before bed, so that you are not hungry at night. Also, try to avoid sugary snacks before bed as they may cause the blood sugar to plummet when you are asleep and may lead to waking.

Ways to relax

Increased cortisol levels due to stress may also affect sleep quality. These levels will improve as the breathing pattern improves and will lead to better quality sleep.

Some people may find progressive muscle relaxation beneficial to help them get to sleep, while others say they find it irritating or not helpful. Progressive muscle relaxation is done while in bed –

you tense and then relax each muscle group in turn, starting at the feet and moving upwards to the legs, thighs, abdomen, upper body and head, face and chin.

If progressive muscle relaxation does not appeal, perhaps guided relaxation, meditation, sleep sounds or sleep music may be beneficial. Apps for these are available, but it's best to try a sample before you buy, as many contain deep-breathing or mouth-breathing exercises. I have found that guided imagery is very effective in helping people to relax and improve their breathing pattern. This is something I implement while using capnometry with clients when they are finding it difficult to relax. A hypothetical trip to the forest, mountains or beach is very relaxing and quickly reduces anxiety levels, as well as creating significant improvements in your breathing pattern and end-tidal carbon dioxide levels.

Your bedroom

Your bedroom should preferably be airy but not cold, ideally around 18 degrees Celsius. The body's temperature drops before sleep and is at its lowest in the early hours of the morning. If you become overheated, you may wake up or semi-wake during the night.

Like Goldilocks, your bed should be just right for you. If you wake up with a backache or feeling stiff all over, consider changing your bed or at least changing your mattress. If you find that you sleep better while on holiday, observe the type of bed you sleep in while you are away. Is it hard or soft or in between? The density of the mattress may be the reason why you are sleeping better and not necessarily the relaxed atmosphere or reduced stress levels while on holiday.

If you associate your bed with anxiety and sleeplessness – and some people do – then consider switching to another bed or even sleeping on the couch for a few nights to help you break that association. I have had several clients who could not sleep in their own bed for a few nights until their breathing improved, following which they were fine returning to it.

If you wake at night with an anxiety or panic attack, sit up and initiate the Controlled Breathing Exercise described in Week 1. When your breathing and heart rates have stabilised, settle down again.

Stop snoring

You may wake yourself up if you snore or you may partially wake up and not recall that you have been snoring, then the next day you may feel fatigued and lack concentration. Snoring is generally due to turbulence and greater volumes of air inhaled through the mouth. Often it is the bed partner who complains that snoring is waking them up or preventing them from sleeping. If you don't know whether you snore or not, perhaps try recording your breathing at night to find out. To avoid snoring:

- Sleep on your side. You are more likely to nose-breathe and therefore reduce the volume of air inhaled.
- Use a couple of pillows under your head so that you are not too flat.
- Check your alignment at night. Your head and body should be in alignment as you sleep on your side. If your head is thrust forward and you are C-shaped while sleeping on your side, your airway will be constricted and this may contribute to turbulence and snoring.

If your breathing pattern during the day is disordered or inefficient, it will continue to be a problem at night and may be even worse at night due to the fact that it's more difficult to breathe while lying down. But the good news is that as you improve your breathing, your sleep will also improve.

The insomnia cycle

You lie awake, mind racing, thinking about all the things you need to do tomorrow and how you really need some sound sleep right now or life will be very challenging. Your partner is asleep within six breaths and you lie there wondering how they do it!

There is a medical term for the length of time it takes to get to sleep: 'sleep latency'. The normal sleep latency is five to ten minutes. Insomnia means lack of sleep or the inability to sleep. Insomnia is a common problem associated with stress, anxiety and over-breathing. Often the worst part of not sleeping well is that anxiety levels increase when we are not able to get to sleep or when we keep waking up and then cannot get back to sleep, with the added stress of knowing that we have to perform and do our work or study as usual the next day.

If this is happening to you, I recommend the following:

- Remind yourself that the body is the 'ultimate machine' and will always look after itself; it will make sure you get enough core sleep to get by. Generally you will make up for lost sleep the following night when the pressure is off.
- Try not to catnap too much during the day or it may interfere with sleep at night.
- Try a meditation or relaxation strategy, as described earlier.

- If you can't get to sleep or if you wake up and you are having trouble getting back to sleep, initiate the Controlled Breathing Exercise described in Week 1 while lying on your side. This will allow you to focus on your breathing and calm a busy or anxious thought pattern as you drift off to sleep.

- Try not to watch the clock – turn it away from your line of vision.

- If you are still awake and if you have been lying awake for twenty minutes or more, get up, have a drink of water, and do some light reading for ten minutes, then go back to bed and try the Controlled Breathing Exercise again.

- If your sleep pattern is really out of kilter, ask your pharmacist about some non-prescription sleep aids as a temporary solution.

- If your sleep pattern is very disordered and you feel sleepy at the wrong time or you lie awake for large portions of the night, you may need to consider visiting your doctor to discuss the possibility of using some melatonin on a temporary basis to help you adjust. A more natural way to reset the body clock is outdoor exposure to daylight earlier in the day. This lets the body know that it is daytime and therefore time to decrease melatonin levels until the light starts to fade at dusk.

As your breathing pattern improves during the daytime and stress levels are reduced, your sleep will also improve.

The best exercise for breathing, sleep and mood

Walk your way to better health and breathing

Believe it or not, walking is the best exercise while retraining the breathing pattern. Walking helps the brain to switch off and calm down. Walking also helps to balance our hormone levels, including adrenaline and cortisol. Even more importantly, walking helps us to increase our carbon dioxide levels – a key requirement to improving the breathing pattern.

When we move or perform any physical exercise such as walking, extra energy is needed, therefore extra carbon dioxide is produced as a result of the energy expended through oxygenation of the cells. Nose-breathing will help you to retain that extra carbon dioxide and allow you to gradually acclimatise to normal carbon dioxide levels.

I recommend that you start a formal routine of daily walking, depending on your fitness level, where you can concentrate on nose-breathing. Be careful to nose-breathe only, while inhaling and exhaling during your walk. The aim is to nose-breathe comfortably, not to raise a sweat or to exercise (although this may happen coincidentally). At this stage it would be preferable to walk on level ground and not attempt stairs or inclines or hills if you are finding it difficult to nose-breathe – these can come later. Of course, if you normally have to climb stairs, do them very slowly, stopping to catch your breath as required, so that you can comfortably nose-breathe.

As hunter-gathers, our ancestors walked most of their day, foraging for food except for the odd run to escape predators or to catch some live prey. We are meant to keep moving, not sit at a desk or stand behind a counter. Numerous studies confirm the benefits of exercise on mood and sleep. Whether you are walking to work or to your car, or hunting and gathering around the supermarket, remind yourself to nose-breathe.

Physical exercise such as walking will help you to:

- de-stress
- stop rumination (going over your worries in your head)
- improve sleep, making it easier to fall asleep and stay asleep
- increase carbon dioxide levels and therefore improve breathing
- improve mood, particularly if you walk in a park or green, leafy area.[2, 3]

Walking may also be as effective in treating depression as drug treatment, according to some studies, but do not reduce or cease any medication without consulting your doctor.

It's best to walk earlier in the day or in the afternoon if possible because when we exercise, we raise endorphin levels, the feel-good hormones that give us a 'high'. These increased levels mean it's best to avoid strenuous exercise too close to bedtime so that you have time to calm down as the levels reduce and get to sleep.

Several studies have shown the benefits of walking. A Stanford University study that shows that walking in a tree-lined area has a recognisable effect on the brain and improves mood has the experts very interested.[4] This study compared two groups who walked for the same duration. One group walked in a green, leafy area and the other in a noisy area next to a highway. The group that walked in the green, leafy area improved their tendency to worry and ruminate, and soothed their minds, while the other group's route had no effect on their moods. The results were confirmed by brain scans and questionnaires. No-one knows exactly why the walk in a leafy area soothed the mind and had a calming effect but it's apparent that a green, leafy area is obviously more calming than a loud, noisy area.

The length of your walk will depend on your fitness level, but this is not a fitness activity as such, it is an exercise aimed at improving your breathing and your ability to retain carbon dioxide. But, of course, regular walking will improve your fitness level. I recommend that you start with around fifteen or twenty minutes daily and gradually work up to thirty minutes daily by the end of the week, depending on your fitness level.

Walking is recommended initially in breathing retraining because you can slow down or stop if you are finding it difficult to nose-breathe. Other forms of exercise such as sports or swimming, or attending the gym, can be too difficult at this stage as you may not be able to nose-breathe throughout. These activities can be done later on if you wish, once you have mastered the art of walking and nose-breathing first. There are some guidelines for this later on in the program.

Remember:

- Nose-breathe gently while walking. Slow down or stop if you can't nose-breathe comfortably.
- Keep your shoulders back, down and relaxed.
- Keep your head straight and in line with your body (not thrust forward).

- Let others do the talking if you are walking with someone else. Talking reduces carbon dioxide levels, which is counterproductive to what we are trying to achieve, i.e. to retain and normalise carbon dioxide levels while walking. Later on, you will learn to nose-breathe while talking.

Too cold, too hot or raining? Walking indoors is also fine in terms of increasing and retaining carbon dioxide. You could try walking in a shopping centre when it's fairly quiet, or even on a treadmill, as long as you are nose-breathing.

Over the next few weeks you can slowly and steadily increase the duration and pace of your daily walk, but ensure that you can comfortably nose-breathe throughout. Slow down or stop if you are finding it difficult or if you can't nose-breathe. If you start to mouth-breathe you may undo all the good work of attempting to raise those carbon dioxide levels.

Improve your carbon dioxide levels

Normalising carbon dioxide levels is an essential part of breathing retraining. By improving breathing we begin to *retain* more carbon dioxide and avoid losing this important gas through over-breathing. Mouth-breathing is the most obvious way we lose carbon dioxide, but there are other ways, so it's wise to be aware of these so that we can continue to improve our carbon dioxide levels. Here are some of the important strategies recommended to improve and retain carbon dioxide while you retrain your breathing pattern. These strategies are just temporary guidelines to be aware of for a few weeks until your breathing improves — they won't be used forever.

IMPORTANT STRATEGIES TO IMPROVE CARBON DIOXIDE LEVELS

Coughing

- Avoid prolonged bouts of coughing. For an irritating tickle, take sips of water or a hot drink.
- If you are in the habit of having prolonged coughing bouts after rising in the morning, be especially careful that you nose-breathe on rising and throughout your shower.
- To stop a 'tickly' cough, cough into your cupped hands and then re-breathe the air containing the exhaled carbon dioxide.

Yawning

- Try to avoid frequent yawning. Learn to yawn through your nose. You can still have a nice stretch and feel the benefit and relaxation.

Yelling/shouting

- Avoid yelling or shouting for the time being – particularly while walking the dog or other activities.

Sneezing

- Avoid prolonged bouts of sneezing. Blow your nose or take sips of water after the first couple of sneezes.

Laughing

- Prolonged 'belly laughing' lowers carbon dioxide levels. While laughing is good for you (it improves the immune system), avoid prolonged belly laughing sessions until your breathing is retrained towards normal.

Sighing/throat clearing

- Be aware of these and avoid.

Wear loose clothing

Many of my clients say they notice that their breathing feels more constricted when they wear fitted or tight clothing. Strangely, they only begin to recognise this *after* they begin their breathing retraining course, which is probably why awareness is so important while improving your breathing pattern. If this happens to you, it would be advisable to wear loose clothing for a few weeks until your breathing improves and you are feeling more comfortable, whether it is for sleeping, walking, exercising or daily living. Avoid wearing anything that constricts the breathing, e.g. ties or tops or anything that is tight around the neck, waist or chest.

Stretches

Do you sit or stand for prolonged periods during the day? Do you feel tension in your back, neck or shoulders? I recommend that you start doing some regular stretches. Stand up and walk around for a couple of minutes every hour or so during the day, particularly if you have a sedentary job or sit in front of a computer for prolonged periods. In addition, do some *gentle* stretches, but be careful to nose-breathe while you stretch. Use the three Ss as you stretch:

- slow
- steady
- smooth.

If you have issues or injuries in your shoulders, neck or back (or other muscle or skeletal issues), take professional advice as to which stretches may be appropriate for you.

Healing/clearing reactions

Occasionally people experience a clearing or healing reaction in the first week or so after commencing breathing retraining. This usually takes the form of a headache or a loss of appetite, fatigue or aching muscles. Some people may find that their nose is stuffy or uncomfortable, others may have a runny nose or increased mucus, while others may find their nasal passages become burning or sore. A burning feeling in the nose or a runny nose or increased mucus indicates that the mucous membranes in the nose are adapting to the increased air flow through the nose, and this will gradually diminish and stop after a few days.

If you experience a healing reaction, bear in mind that these reactions are temporary and that they are a good sign, as they mean that your body is adapting to an improving breathing pattern. However, if it becomes too uncomfortable, ease off the breathing retraining exercises for a day or two and then resume slowly.

Consider adding unrefined sea salt or ocean salt to your food to taste – instead of the free-flowing processed salt. This will help to ensure that your mineral intake is improved, which will in turn help to buffer (balance) slight shifts in blood pH that may occur during breathing retraining. In addition, ensure that you have adequate minerals in your diet in the form of fruit, vegetables and nuts.

You may notice that you are yawning more frequently this week and possibly next week. This is part of the body's response to slight increases in carbon dioxide levels. The respiratory centre in the brain monitors our carbon dioxide levels. Yawning or sighing is a normal reaction to slight alterations (improvements) in carbon dioxide levels. When people who have been over-breathing experience slight increases in carbon dioxide, just by nose-breathing or breathing more gently, the body sometimes responds by increasing yawning in order to decrease levels and maintain the status quo. Yawning at this stage is actually a good sign and it is temporary. Learn to yawn through your nose to retain carbon dioxide, and in a few days the yawning will become a thing of the past as you adjust to normalised carbon dioxide levels.

WEEK 2: BREATHING RETRAINING CHECKLIST	
ACTIVITIES	☐ **Walk**: start a daily walk while nose-breathing only, as recommended. ☐ **Wear loose clothing**. ☐ **Stretch**: stand up and do some gentle stretches every hour or two during the day while gently nose-breathing. ☐ Consider adding **unrefined sea salt** to your food to taste as suggested. ☐ Complete your **daily diary**.
BREATHING	☐ Gently **nose-breathe** at all times. ☐ **Improve** your carbon dioxide levels; monitor your breathing and implement the strategies as listed.
POSTURE	☐ Be aware of your posture throughout the day and adopt an **upright but relaxed posture**.
SYMPTOMS	☐ Use the **Controlled Breathing Exercise** described in Week 1 at the first sign of anxiety and panic attacks.
SLEEP	☐ Start a bedtime **routine**: unwind with quiet time, lights and sounds down, read, play soft music. ☐ **Avoid** electronic screens in the hour before bedtime. ☐ **Avoid** caffeine, alcohol, a large meal and strenuous exercise before bed. ☐ **Sleep** *only* on your side. ☐ **Sleep** with your mouth closed; nose-breathe while sleeping.

CHAPTER 19

Week 3: Eat, drink, breathe

It's all in your mind ... or maybe it's all in your gut?

Aims and objectives:

- Learn more advanced breathing retraining exercises.
- Discover the best food and drink to help improve your breathing pattern.
- Discover some lifestyle strategies to help improve breathing and symptoms.
- Learn how to deal with challenging situations.

Advanced breathing retraining exercises

Short Breathing Pause Exercise

Now that you are more comfortable with nose-breathing and you realise the importance of increasing carbon dioxide levels towards normal, the following exercise can be done a maximum of three times a day, spread out over the day. If you find that this exercise induces anxiety, avoid it at this stage. For those who are ready, however, this exercise will help increase your carbon dioxide levels and improve your breathing further. You will need a stopwatch, which you should be able to find on your mobile phone.

- Sit on an upright chair (not a lounge chair) and adopt correct posture.
- Keeping your mouth closed, take a *normal* breath in through your nose, then breathe out through your nose.
- Deliberately hold your breath after exhalation (or hold your nose, if you like) for three to five seconds – *not* more than this.
- Keep your mouth closed and breathe in again gently through your *nose*.
- Nose-breathe gently for a minute or two.
- Repeat this exercise.

You may find that three-second pauses are more comfortable to begin with, and over time these can be increased to five seconds. Avoid mouth-breathing or loud breathing; this exercise – like all the breathing exercises in this book – should feel comfortable at all times. Don't be tempted to take longer pauses or repeat this exercise more than three times a day because it may cause headaches or increase anxiety if you are sensitive to increasing carbon dioxide levels.

The Reading Exercise

As we speak, carbon dioxide levels are quickly depleted, particularly when we are already over-breathing. Being able to control those carbon dioxide levels is very important. Speaking is one of the activities where many people tend to mouth-breathe and therefore may over-breathe, often needing to cough or gulp air mid-sentence. Sometimes gulping air while speaking is one of the clues to over-breathing. When I ask people a question while assessing their breathing pattern with capnometry, they can see how quickly their carbon dioxide levels are reduced when they reply. This reduction in carbon dioxide levels while we speak is normal, but for some people who already have reduced carbon dioxide levels due to over-breathing, speaking can actually *increase* anxiety. I recommend that you use the reading exercise to retrain your breathing pattern while speaking. This will help to reduce anxiety as well as retain carbon dioxide. People such as teachers, or those who sing or play a wind instrument, or who are on the phone a lot or have to speak or make presentations as part of their work find this exercise particularly useful.

The reading exercise that follows is a simple way of controlling and slowing down the speech pattern a little, and can make a significant difference in reducing anxiety, getting rid of that spaced-out feeling and helping you to concentrate and think more clearly. The exercise involves *reading out loud* for just two or three minutes each day, but as usual, there is a catch: you are only allowed to nose-breathe while you read. First, inhale gently through your nose, then read a few words, then inhale again through your nose and read a few more words, breaking up the sentences while inhaling as if there were commas everywhere. Don't worry about the out-breath: your speech *is* the out-breath. Just use a conversational tone and don't try to project your voice too loudly at the start.

This exercise is not as easy as it sounds and your reading may feel disjointed and unnatural at first, but it does get easier with practice. The reading exercise is very helpful for reducing that gulping-for-air pattern many people who are over-breathing adopt while speaking.

I have also seen this reading exercise routine work really well to reduce stammering.

You have to be able to walk before you can run!

Last week, you began your daily walk while nose-breathing. This week, if appropriate for your fitness level, try increasing your pace a little while maintaining nose-breathing. Once you are comfortable with this, you could try interval training. Every two or three minutes during your walk, try walking a little faster or jog for one minute while you continue to nose-breathe. This may feel a little difficult at first, so take it slowly. Avoid making yourself too breathless; your breathing should be comfortable, although it will be a little deeper. With time it becomes easier. You could also take the stairs (slowly) as part of your nose-breathing exercise routine.

Generally, it takes around a month or more to be able to jog slowly and predominantly nose-breathe for twenty minutes. It may take a little longer for some people. The old saying 'You have to be able to walk before you can run' is very apt here!

Always consult your doctor before starting any
exercise program, including any mentioned
in this book. All exercises and activities
need to be within your fitness capacity
and under the guidance of your doctor.

Over the next few weeks you may want to progress to more active physical exercise. If you are constantly anxious or if you tend to ruminate, you may find that physical exercise such as walking or jogging is a great way to clear your head, blow away those anxieties and worries, and make you feel better. You may also get an endorphin rush when you do vigorous physical exercise. Although carbon dioxide levels may increase tenfold while exercising, arterial carbon dioxide levels are regulated and maintained within a precise range.

This book cannot provide all the information required for every exercise and sports program. Therefore, all exercise strategies need to be within your fitness capacity and under the guidance of a trainer or your doctor.

Take time out

Every day, try to take just five minutes to sit and reflect and gently nose-breathe, preferably outdoors. This will help to calm your anxiety and improve stress levels, while improving your breathing pattern. Don't try to order your thoughts or analyse; just allow your thoughts to drift as they come and go. This kind of reverie or daydreaming will help to slow down those busy thoughts and help to improve breathing.

Food and nutrition issues

In practice, I have found that most people experiencing anxiety
and panic symptoms are very conscientious about eating a
healthy diet. However, if you are considering making significant
changes to your diet or supplementing with probiotics, or if
you have IBS, it would be prudent to consult your healthcare
professional or a nutritionist.

Over-breathing may be associated with poor food choices.
Over-eating (particularly a diet high in animal protein), or a
diet high in sugar or starches, or an unbalanced diet that is high
in processed foods or a diet with additives like food colouring,
flavour enhancers or preservatives may be contributing factors.
In hunter-gatherer societies there was no processed food, and if
they wanted sweetness, they ate berries and fruits in season or
risked getting stung by bees if they raided their hives.

If you would like to lose weight (or gain weight) I advise
you not to become too focused on this issue while in the initial
stages of your breathing retraining program. It's better to
focus on one thing at a time – and improving the breathing
pattern and sleep are a priority. Once these are achieved, you
can then start to focus more on weight issues, if needed. In my
experience, a person's weight (whether under- or overweight)
tends to stabilise towards normal when their breathing pattern
and their sleep improve. If you are overweight or underweight,
have blood-sugar issues, diabetes or other food-related problems,
please consult your doctor or a nutritionist before making major
changes to your diet.

General guidelines on food while retraining breathing are
provided in Figure 19.1.

FIGURE 19.1: GUIDELINES ON FOOD
WHILE RETRAINING BREATHING

1. Eat only when you are hungry; stop eating when you are full.
2. Eat in moderation and avoid over-eating. In order to digest food, the metabolism increases, and this includes the breathing rate and the heart rate. Over-eating may raise the breathing rate and volume.
3. Avoid eating excessive amounts of animal protein.
4. Try eating smaller, more frequent meals until your breathing improves.
5. Add unprocessed sea salt or ocean salt to your food to taste, instead of the processed free-flowing variety.
6. Avoid dips in blood sugar: don't skip meals. Decreases in blood sugar may increase anxiety and lead to feeling spaced out or to a panic attack.
7. Eat balanced meals. Include plenty of non-starchy vegetables and salads. Include a wide variety of colourful vegetables, especially green leafy vegetables.
8. Avoid added sugar, food additives, preservatives, flavour enhancers or colouring in food and beverages.
9. Eat naturally; that means eating unprocessed foods that come from nature – not from a package. If Great-grandma wouldn't recognise them, avoid eating them.
10. Include unsalted nuts and seeds in your diet to help boost mineral levels.
11. Take time to sit down to eat, preferably with your family or friends. Socialising is a great way to alleviate stress and anxiety. Avoid rushing your meals or eating on the go.
12. Chew your food carefully with your mouth closed. This avoids swallowing air, which may contribute to bloating.
13. Try to avoid eating a large meal within two hours of bedtime; it puts a strain on your digestion and may affect your breathing and your sleep.
14. Start to reduce caffeine, especially in the hours before bed.
15. If you like a drink, enjoy a glass of alcohol but don't overdo it, particularly close to bedtime.
16. Drink water rather than cola, soft drinks, fizzy drinks or sports drinks.
17. If you keep waking up at night, avoid late-night snacks of meat, cheese or dairy products before bed. Some people don't tolerate dairy very well, and they wake up during the night if they eat dairy foods close to bedtime. You could try avoiding dairy products for a few days (or at least for a few hours before bed) and monitor your response. You could also look at low blood sugar as a possible culprit (see overleaf for details). See your doctor if waking persists.

Blood-sugar issues

'Sugar is toxic' has become the mantra of many food and nutrition experts. As a society we are only now beginning to realise just how damaging and unhealthy excessive sugar consumption is, and there is now increasing evidence of an association between excessive sugar consumption and the incidence of obesity and type 2 diabetes.

Sugar in small quantities is not toxic; it is contained naturally in fruit and even in some vegetables. But many processed foods and drinks contain huge amounts of *added* sugar, which spike the blood sugar and cause health issues. Today, sugar is not only plentiful; it is hiding in many of the foodstuffs we eat regularly, some of which we may not even associate with sugar. Even a small pot of sweetened yoghurt – which many consider a healthy food – or a 'healthy' muesli bar may contain as many as four or five teaspoons of sugar.

Excessive sugar consumption, processed food and reduced fibre may contribute to microbiome imbalances and gut issues. Excessive sugar also hypes us up and increases the heart and breathing rates, putting the body into overdrive, which means you may find it difficult to sleep. In turn, an imbalance in the gut microbiome may lead to constant cravings for sugar or starchy food, as the 'bad' bugs in the gut cry out for their daily fix.

The use of sugary foods to help calm down or decrease anxiety or panic symptoms may need to be tackled carefully, as a reduction in sugar intake may temporarily increase anxiety symptoms. In these instances, a gradual reduction in sugar (beginning with no added sugar) over several days or over a week or two may be necessary, while at the same time adopting the recommended strategies and techniques to improve the breathing pattern.

In general, adopting a diet of natural, unprocessed food is recommended as the best option to stabilise blood sugar levels and avoid the highs and lows that accompany processed and sugary food and drinks. Don't be fooled by claims that everything from a juicer is healthy. Fruit juice is a highly processed drink, therefore drinking lots of fruit juice is not a healthy option. Fruit juice is high in fructose, a type of sugar found in fruit. Consider the number of oranges in a glass of orange juice – possibly five or six. Most of us could not eat that number of oranges in one session. Excessive amounts of fructose may spike the blood sugar and trigger fluctuations in blood sugar levels. Whole fruit in moderation is preferable to juice. Just think about our hunter-gatherer ancestors: they would have eaten seasonal whole fruit when available; fruit juice was not on the menu.

If you suspect you may have hypoglycaemia or low blood sugar:

- consult your healthcare professional
- eat frequent and regular meals
- avoid added sugars
- avoid processed foods (which usually have added sugar)
- avoid fruit juice, eating a small amount of whole fruit instead
- have low-GI snacks
- avoid alcohol.

Food and sleep issues

For some people, poor sleep may be associated with food intolerance or sensitivity. I recall the story of Jason, a young man who'd had problems with insomnia and who woke several times at night, every night. Jason had never slept well from around the age of twelve, and in his twenties, he decided to do a breathing retraining course because of asthma. A couple of weeks after the course I spoke with Jason on the phone. He reported that he was doing fine and didn't need his asthma puffer. When I asked if his sleep had improved, his answer was surprising. 'Yes,' he said, 'I found out what was causing the problem!'

I was curious, so I asked what it was.

'It was that big bowl of ice-cream I had every night before bed!' Jason loved ice-cream, and from the age of twelve he had treated himself to a bowl every night. It was not until he did a breathing retraining course that he found out that the dairy and sugar in the ice-cream could be affecting his breathing pattern and his sleep.

We all love chocolate

Chocolate is thought to trigger the feel-good hormone, serotonin, which (as well as the taste) is probably why most of us love chocolate. But chocolate is also high in fat and sugar, as well as containing the stimulants theobromine and caffeine, which, if eaten in excess, may increase the heart rate and therefore increase the breathing rate. Chocolate can cause palpitations or insomnia in some people, so it's best to avoid eating it before bed if you are sensitive to caffeine. Also, the sugar in chocolate may cause blood sugar to spike and later drop, which may contribute to waking during the night with low blood sugar levels – or possibly panic symptoms – in susceptible individuals.

The good news is that chocolate contains magnesium, which helps us to relax, as well as antioxidants, which may protect us from cardiovascular disease and cancer. For these reasons many experts advise that eating a little dark chocolate now and then may be beneficial, although the jury is still out to some extent.

If you love chocolate, a little dark chocolate (one or two squares) containing 85 per cent cocoa fat is acceptable occasionally. But even this contains added sugar or it would be too bitter for our tastebuds.

Lifestyle issues

For many people, a glass of wine or a beer is just one of life's pleasures, and I have to agree with that philosophy! However, drinking alcohol in excessive amounts is sometimes a coping mechanism people adopt when their stress, anxiety or panic symptoms become overwhelming. Alcohol depresses the nervous system and some people may use it as a crutch to help them to feel calm – temporarily. Unfortunately, we can develop a tolerance for alcohol, so over time more is needed to have the same effect.

Also, alcohol may worsen chronic anxiety in some people and may cause a dependence to develop. In these circumstances, overuse can also lead to depression. I'm not knocking alcohol per se – a glass of wine or beer, or a serving of spirits, can be relaxing and enjoyable – but if you are overdoing it and having more than one or two serves of alcohol per day, you may be using it as a coping mechanism and you may need to consider reducing the amount you consume.

Also, if you do like a glass of wine or a beer, that's fine, but try not to have alcohol within two hours of bedtime. Drinking alcohol before bed may:

- worsen your breathing pattern
- cause dehydration
- wreak havoc on your blood sugar
- disrupt your sleep cycle and prevent you from having refreshing sleep.

While alcohol may help you to get to sleep initially, the chances are there will be a rebound effect and you will wake after around ninety minutes, just when you should be going into a cycle of the essential REM sleep (rapid eye movement, or dream sleep). You may then find it difficult to get back to sleep or you may have a restless night. Refreshing sleep is critical for reducing stress, anxiety and panic, and for improving your breathing pattern.

Excessive consumption of tea and coffee may also be an issue and may increase your breathing rate. Many of us enjoy a cup of tea or coffee during the day; it's our go-to drink as a pick-me-up or source of energy. And there is evidence that tea and coffee in moderation may be good for us. According to some sources, coffee consumption in moderation may be associated with lower early mortality risks.[1] But the caffeine in tea and coffee is a stimulant and if used in excess it may stimulate the breathing pattern and the heart rate, something we are trying to avoid while retraining our breathing. Some people get palpitations after drinking coffee, and in these people caffeine may need to be significantly reduced or even eliminated. Caffeine is also found in cola, some fizzy drinks, and sports and energy drinks. These can make us feel hyped and full of energy, but they may also increase anxiety by raising the breathing pattern and heart rate.

Studies suggest that caffeine can remain in the blood for as long as eight hours; therefore, if you don't sleep well it would make sense to avoid caffeine drinks in the afternoon and evening in order to improve sleep.

You may have developed a physical dependence on caffeine; if so, it's important to reduce your caffeine intake very slowly. Perhaps make a withdrawal schedule showing how much you're drinking and how you intend to reduce the amount until you reach one cup of coffee or a couple of cups of weak tea per day. Cutting them out all at once may increase anxiety, so my advice is to take it slowly and gradually decrease these over time. Reducing caffeine gradually in this way may also help to avoid withdrawal symptoms such as headaches and fatigue.

For the average person, I recommend avoiding sports drinks or at least taking the time to read the label to ensure they are a healthy choice. Some may look healthy or be touted as 'all natural', but if you read the label carefully you may find that they contain high quantities of sugar, caffeine or guarana (another stimulant), preservatives, additives or food colouring.

Water is the best option if you need a cold drink. You can make it more interesting with ice, fresh mint and lemon slices. Some sliced kiwi fruit or strawberry will also make it feel special.

Cigarettes

Cigarettes are also used by some people as a way to relax and as a coping mechanism. I prefer not to lecture my clients about cutting down on cigarettes – they already know how damaging smoking is. Smoking is one of the hardest addictions to overcome. However, smokers may not be aware that smoking can actually reinforce over-breathing habits through inhaling and exhaling more deeply as the person smokes. If you are struggling, I advise you to see your health professional for advice or help on quitting smoking.

Dreams

Some of my clients have commented that they hadn't dreamt in ages until their breathing pattern started to improve. We all dream, so what they actually mean is that they don't recall their dreams. Or they may not be getting sufficient REM (rapid eye movement) sleep, which is the stage of sleep needed for dreaming. It is thought that we consolidate memories during REM sleep. I like to think of it a bit like a computer filing things into the right place and storing them away.

Other clients may say they have had frightening dreams before their breathing retraining course. Frightening dreams are one of the characteristics of over-breathing (see Chapter 4, Table 4.1).

Rarely, some of my clients say they have started to have frightening dreams or more vivid dreams as their breathing improves, and this may be a bit scary. They may wonder if they are doing something wrong or if they are dragging up issues from the past. If this happens, it doesn't mean that you are doing anything wrong. It's a temporary thing and is a normal part of recovery. Frightening dreams in this circumstance may be part of our way of dealing with change and trying to compartmentalise or place things into the right boxes, so that we can move on.

Coping with challenges

Does the thought of going for a job interview strike fear in your heart? Or perhaps other challenges, such as meeting new people, making a speech, giving a presentation, doing an examination, or coping with a difficult boss give you butterflies in the stomach? These are stressful situations for almost everyone. We need to accept that there may be some stress as we move forwards; however, there are some strategies that may help you to cope with the stress, as far as your breathing pattern is concerned.

If you are faced with an important or challenging event, I recommend some extra strategies to minimise anxiety. A little adrenaline is okay – it keeps us focused – but excess adrenaline can make us feel anxious, spaced or shaky and may lead to reduced blood sugar (hypoglycaemia).

Before the challenging situation

Ensure that you become thoroughly acquainted with the Controlled Breathing Exercise described in Week 1. If you feel anxious, do not be tempted to take deep breaths to help calm you down. If you are anxious, your breathing will already be deeper and the volume increased, or you may be shallow-breathing, rapidly breathing or gulping air – even though you may feel you cannot get enough air. You do not need to do deep breathing; instead concentrate on slow, comfortable and *controlled* nose-breathing.

Take time to do some of the Controlled Breathing Exercise routine. No-one can tell if you are doing this exercise. You could also try walking around as you gently nose-breathe.

Another point to bear in mind if you have an important presentation or speech coming up is to avoid alcohol before you speak. Combining alcohol with anxiety does not make for a clear head, so it's best to avoid alcohol in these situations.

When we are anxious, extra insulin is produced and this in turn may lead to hypoglycaemia or low blood sugar, causing us to feel light-headed, spaced out, shaky and anxious. By eating a low glycaemic index (GI) snack before a challenging event, you will help counteract any excess insulin and help keep a clear head. Low-GI snacks include a banana or some nuts, or avocado or hummus on wholegrain crackers. Eating a low-GI snack five or ten minutes before a challenging event will ensure that the food will be metabolised more slowly and will therefore keep your blood sugar stable.

Avoid eating sugary snacks or drinks to help calm you down. These will spike your blood sugar quickly and make it come crashing down again, which could make you even more anxious or spaced out.

WEEK 3: BREATHING RETRAINING CHECKLIST	
ACTIVITIES	❑ Continue your **daily walk** as described last week and, if you can comfortably nose-breathe, try walking a little faster or walking on an incline or include some stairs or steps as part of your walk. ❑ **Start to reduce stimulants and sugar**, including coffee, strong tea, colas and sports drinks containing caffeine, sugar or guarana. ❑ Start to implement the **food and nutrition** guidelines in Figure 19.1. ❑ Start the **Short Breathing Pause Exercise** as described. ❑ Practise the **Reading Exercise** for two or three minutes each day as described. ❑ Take **time out** for five minutes each day just to sit and daydream. ❑ Continue with some *gentle* **stretches** now and then during the day while nose-breathing. ❑ Complete your **daily diary**.
BREATHING	❑ When moving, walking or exercising, continue to make gentle **nose-breathing** a habit.
POSTURE	❑ As usual, be aware of your posture throughout the day and adopt an upright but relaxed posture.
SYMPTOMS	❑ Continue to use the **Controlled Breathing Exercise** described in Week 1 if you are experiencing symptoms.
SLEEP	❑ Continue to **sleep** only on your side; sleep with your mouth closed. ❑ Check your **alignment** at night if you snore or if you keep waking up with symptoms.

CHAPTER 20

Week 4: De-stress, boost confidence

Imagine telling a caveman he needs to improve his work–life balance!

Aims and objectives:

- Learn the seven steps to de-stress.
- Discover twenty ways to boost confidence and self-esteem.
- Learn how to increase exercise on the Nose-breathing Pyramid.
- Start to work on no-go zones or avoidance issues if necessary.

Someone once said that the secret to a happy marriage is low expectations (Warren Buffett, American investments guru, perhaps). Very apt, but not really all that surprising! The greater the expectations, the greater the pressure; the greater the pressure, the greater the stress; and the greater the stress on a relationship, the greater the possibility of separation or divorce. The same formula could be applied to life in general, and in particular to people struggling with anxiety and panic symptoms.

People who are already stressed need less pressure, not more. That is why I have tried to make the strategies suggested in this book practical, appealing and doable within the average person's schedule.

It seems that each generation grows up with different life expectations. Some of us may have grown up with the self-entitlement expectations of the Me generation of Baby Boomers, while others may belong to the post–Baby Boomer Gen X, who are said to be 'self-starters' and more inclined to pursue life balance. The Millennials or Gen Y were brought up in a digital age and are said to have been raised in a more sheltered way (driven to school, etc.) but are more competitive. These are all generalisations, of course. Most of us (and that includes many people experiencing anxiety and panic) struggle with high expectations, whether self-imposed or imposed by others. Trying to balance home life, social life, relationships and career appears to be a rather good idea.

But if you think about it, there is no such thing as the perfect life balance, and the expectation of such may put extra pressure on already stressed and pressured individuals. Imagine telling a caveman that he needs to improve his work–life balance! It would be ludicrous! Basically, we are survivors, and we survived long enough to procreate by keeping safe. In many situations, striving for the perfect life balance is akin to striving for the impossible.

Having a nice balance of work, rest and play is just an aspiration. So avoid putting extra pressure on yourself and trying to attain perfection, i.e. the impossible. Think of yourself as a survivor and do whatever it takes to get you through. Of course, do so without causing harm to yourself or anyone else. During this period of breathing retraining, be kind to yourself and try not to place unrealistic expectations on yourself. Once your breathing pattern has improved and your symptoms are not so troublesome, you will be able to see things more clearly and – if you feel the need – set realistic and achievable goals.

Seven steps to de-stress

The greatest contributor to over-breathing is stress. In figure 20.1 you will see some simple steps that I have found have helped my clients to de-stress. These don't all have to be completed at once. In fact, it's better if you do them one or two at a time. You don't need to put yourself under extra pressure! Gradually adopting some of these steps will help you to de-stress, and will help you to be able to withstand stress in the long term without becoming overwhelmed. The first two strategies, improving breathing and improving sleep, are the most important, so once you have these under control, you could start on some of the other steps as necessary.

Stress is the greatest contributor to over-breathing, and the over-breathing habit perpetuates and contributes to anxiety and panic symptoms.

If you lead a very full life and you feel confident, that's great; stress may not be an issue for you. But I have found that most people who experience anxiety and panic symptoms are stressed, sometimes without even being aware of their stress levels, and have had their confidence gradually eroded by their symptoms – so some form of de-stressing is necessary, depending on the person. As mentioned, not all people are alike. For example, some people may find meditation irritating and however hard they try, they just don't get it, while others find it a useful way to de-stress. It's a question of horses for courses. When you feel ready, you can begin to work on steps 3 to 7.

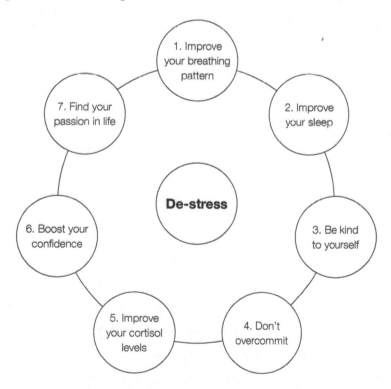

Figure 20.1: Seven steps to de-stress

Step 1 – Improve your breathing pattern

If you have been following the program from Week 1, by this stage you are probably already feeling the benefits of improving your breathing pattern. Patience is key here, particularly if you have been over-breathing for a long time (months or years) or if your condition was severe. It may take a few weeks (or more) to achieve the full benefits.

Step 2 – Improve your sleep

Lack of refreshing sleep can leave us feeling very vulnerable, and we are more likely to feel stressed and overwhelmed by our workload or because of other issues. In Weeks 1 and 2, I have suggested some strategies to help you to get a better night's sleep, and combining these strategies with improving your breathing pattern will help to improve your sleep and may assist you to feel better and to withstand stress more readily.

Improving sleep will also lead to improvements in cortisol levels and a sense of calm.

Step 3 – Be kind to yourself

We all need to unwind and de-stress, and this is particularly important if you are recovering from anxiety and panic symptoms. This week, consider introducing some (achievable!) stress-reducing or relaxation strategies into your life. You can do these alone or with friends or family. The good news is they don't need to be expensive or time-consuming.

Depending on your circumstances, I recommend that you consider doing something just for you, whether it is taking some time out, taking up a hobby or becoming involved in your community. Being part of a tribe helps us to feel better about ourselves, and more secure. You don't need to devote hours of your time – the important thing is to get started. But don't overcommit: try one achievable aim at a time.

Some suggestions are:

- Take time out with friends or join a group. See online or ask at your local library or community centre about men's groups, women's groups, history groups, speakers' groups, meditation groups, book clubs or walking groups. Some libraries have a newcomers' folder, which lists different activities you might be interested in joining.
- Take up a hobby or course that you'd love to do. We all need to live in the moment and calm down those busy thoughts to reduce stress. Depending on your preference, something creative such as writing, pottery or other forms of art may appeal.
- Volunteer – if you have the time, but don't overcommit. Generally, libraries have a list of organisations needing volunteers.
- If you are sedentary, then perhaps something like tai chi, yoga or a fitness class may be helpful. It's important to be able to nose-breathe while you engage in any active sport or hobby. Yoga, chi gong or tai chi, which focus on 'controlled' breathing through the nose, can help to induce calm. Avoid any activity that encourages deep breathing or mouth-breathing.

Before committing to a course, I recommend that you call the instructor or tutor and ask what type of breathing is involved for activities such as yoga, meditation, tai chi or fitness programs.

If you are advised to take deep breaths, or to breathe through the mouth (either in or out, or a combination of mouth-breathing and nose-breathing), this is not the class for you – it may increase breathing or reinforce a disordered breathing pattern, which is something to be avoided.

Step 4 – Don't overcommit

Assertiveness is important here. Saying no is a practice many of us do not feel comfortable with. Becoming assertive will help you to become more comfortable with saying no and feeling good about yourself. Assertiveness is different from aggressiveness. Assertiveness means respecting the rights of others while clearly asserting your rights as a person without anger or intimidation. It doesn't mean, however, that you always get whatever you want! Aggressiveness, on the other hand, may be associated with manipulative behaviour or with threats, anger and intimidation, or with tactics that do not respect your rights or the rights of others.

Saying no

When invited to go somewhere or to help out, do you automatically say 'yes' to people without thinking? We are all guilty of this at some stage or another. Whether it's due to fear of offending, fear of rejection, or striving to be all things to all people – or even being 'nice' to people – over-commitment increases stress levels.

Saying yes without looking at your schedule or consulting your loved ones may impose more stress in the long run. If you are invited to do something or go somewhere – even if it's something you really want to do – get into the habit of not saying yes straightaway. I have said yes on a number of occasions, only to find that the event clashed with something important like a family holiday. It's sometimes time-consuming and embarrassing to have to call and reschedule, especially if the person who requested help is relying on you. So always check your schedule *before* you commit. It may be prudent to respond to an invitation or a request by saying, 'Thank you, that sounds great/really interesting. Let me look at my/our schedule and I'll get back to you.'

The same applies to work situations. Allowing yourself to be overloaded will only lead to resentment and even more stress. If asked to do something you know will increase your workload significantly, point out in your best friendly, casual voice: 'I've still got X, Y and Z to work on, so it will be a while before I can get around to it.' Or even a straight: 'I'm not able to take that on right now, due to other commitments [and describe these other commitments].' You could ask if there is a completion deadline to see if you can realistically fit it in with your work schedule.

Learning to say no is an art, and you can find more information on this topic in books on self-esteem and assertiveness in your local library or online. For some people, learning to say no politely and courteously is not easy. If you have trouble, consider doing a course on assertiveness training. Some free courses on this topic are available online.

Step 5 – Improve your cortisol levels

The hormone cortisol is usually increased in times of stress. This increase can lead to sleep issues, which in turn may increase breathing and exacerbate anxiety or panic. But there are ways to reduce and counteract increases in cortisol. Feeling connected and interacting positively with others, physical contact and being part of a community can help to reduce anxiety and normalise cortisol levels. This will help to improve the balance between the sympathetic nervous system (fight-or-flight) and the parasympathetic nervous system (rest-and-digest) and allow us to achieve a sense of calm.

Here are some of the methods to consider:

- Ensure you get enough refreshing sleep (discussed in detail in Week 3).
- Engage with others socially in a positive way.
- Listen to music – several studies show that listening to music for half an hour lowers cortisol.
- Have a massage.
- Walk (while nose-breathing, of course!).
- Laugh – but see the caution in Week 2 about prolonged belly laughing at an early stage of your program.
- Dance or exercise – also very good, but you need to be able to nose-breathe while doing these activities. Therefore, if you are unable to nose-breathe predominantly throughout, strenuous exercise is best left until later.

Depending on your personal preference, introduce some of these activities into your life on a regular basis. For example, listening to soothing music could be done before bed most nights as an unwinding or relaxation strategy. Treat yourself to a massage now and then if you like massage. Perhaps your partner would be willing to give you a massage occasionally if funds are not available for a professional massage therapist. You will know which activities are best for you if you feel calm and relaxed afterwards.

As mentioned previously, meditation or relaxation can be helpful to induce sleep, and improved sleep will help to normalise cortisol levels. Some people may find it difficult to meditate, but they are able to unwind with a relaxation exercise or with guided relaxation.

Some of my clients find it difficult to relax initially. It can seem as if they are experiencing everything (including breathing) in fast-forward and it's difficult to calm down. If you find that meditation is difficult as it may be hard to switch off those busy thoughts, perhaps try soft music or time out instead.

When you have become more comfortable with nose-breathing while sitting or walking, other exercise such as dancing or a fitness regimen may be initiated, but be careful to take it slowly at first and nose-breathe only during the exercise. Belly dancing is a great way to de-stress (and become fit) if you can find a good teacher.

These strategies don't have to cost much. For example, dancing to music in your lounge room will help you to become accustomed to moving while nose-breathing, and at the same time will help to make you feel better, sleep better, and normalise those cortisol levels. But don't attempt any strenuous exercise in the hours before bed or you may become too energised to sleep.

Step 6 – Boost your confidence

'Two men looked out from prison bars; one saw mud, the other saw stars.'

Dale Carnegie

Are you a glass-half-empty or glass-half-full type of person? Do you see yourself and the world in a positive light?

Rest assured that you did nothing, either consciously or subconsciously, to initiate your anxiety or panic symptoms.

If you are being hard on yourself or blaming yourself (or others) for increased stress levels, anxiety and panic symptoms, or for not being tough enough to cope, you may need to think again. Rest assured that you did nothing, either consciously or subconsciously, to initiate your anxiety or panic symptoms. No-one would willingly wish for or bring anxiety, panic symptoms or over-breathing on themselves, and I am always amazed at how resilient my clients are despite their anxiety and panic symptoms. They are invariably hard-working and very conscientious people.

If you have begun to view your stress, anxiety or panic as a weakness, perhaps it's time to reassess. Seeing yourself in a more positive light will help. And developing some compassion for yourself as well as others is important in achieving a sense of calm and wellbeing. You may be thinking that your body has failed you or let you down in some way, because of the stress, anxiety or panic symptoms you have experienced. On the contrary, the body does everything for a reason, and while you might not have been aware of it, your body has been doing its job and trying to keep you safe!

At some stage, increased stress levels probably caused your brain to perceive that you were unsafe, and we can deduce that the over-breathing habit and the ensuing symptoms were protective, keeping you alert or vigilant for signs of danger. Far from failing you, your brain and your body may have become *overprotective*. The important thing now is that you are doing something positive to improve your breathing pattern and your symptoms by undertaking this program. I recommend that you become your own best friend and take care of yourself. Making time for yourself is important, particularly if you lead a very busy life.

When we have high stress levels or anxiety and panic symptoms it's difficult to enjoy life's pleasures. Sometimes the best we can do is try to get through each day hour by hour, or simply exist, hoping that things will change.

Now that things *are* changing, getting back in touch with the pleasures of life as you improve your breathing pattern is important. These are a few of my recommendations, but of course it's fine to become your own advocate and think of other suggestions from your perspective:

- Live in the moment. The past is history and the future is unknown. Therefore, the only thing we have is this moment – and this moment will never come again.
- Take time to enjoy and appreciate the company of family and friends, or the current event or activity.
- Take time to slow down and smell the roses – literally and metaphorically.
- Give yourself permission to think and act like a hedonist occasionally. Give yourself a treat for having done the breathing retraining exercises: a special outing, a nice meal, organise a massage or even take a warm, relaxing bath.

- Take time to savour and enjoy your meals. Concentrate on quality foods and avoid fast food or processed foods. Reward yourself with a little dark chocolate occasionally. When your breathing has improved and you are sleeping better and feeling less stressed, you will be able to take better care of yourself.
- Improve your posture, if needed. Consider doing some sessions on the Alexander Technique (which focuses on correct posture) or find a book on this topic.

Twenty ways to boost self-confidence

If you feel that your confidence needs a boost, then you may want to consider some of the recommendations in Figure 20.2. You may be able to implement some of these suggestions straightaway, but don't try to tackle all of them at once. Acts of kindness or altruism and being thoughtful about others bring their own rewards. Even small random acts of kindness (without expecting a thank you) make us feel better and more in tune with the world around us.

When you are ready, choose one or two of the following Twenty Ways to Boost Confidence (Figure 20.2) each week and work through the list over the next few weeks. You are probably well on your way with the first step.

FIGURE 20.2: TWENTY WAYS TO BOOST CONFIDENCE

1. Improve your breathing pattern (hopefully, you are well on the way with this step).
2. Get enough rest and sleep. You will see the world, and yourself, in a more positive light.
3. Improve your nutrition. By now, you will have already started to

improve your health by following the strategies recommended in this book.

4. Engage in your passion in life, i.e. find something you love doing and that you are good at and spend some time on that activity.
5. Become more altruistic and help others.
6. Save some time and energy for yourself.
7. Become assertive: take control of your life and learn to say no.
8. Don't allow others to set your agenda in life.
9. Take time out or take holidays or short breaks.
10. Spend time with genuine friends.
11. Take a trip to a new and inspiring location.
12. Learn a new skill or take up a new hobby. It doesn't have to cost much; free courses are often available in your community, at your library or on the internet.
13. Try to give a genuine compliment to someone every day: your loved ones, your friends, or even to strangers.
14. Stay clear of negative people: they will always try to drag you down with them and may affect your mood.
15. Think positively and you will attract positive people into your life.
16. Be grateful for what you have – there are always others less fortunate.
17. Limit the amount of time spent in the virtual world and spend more time in the real world.
18. Live in the moment – this moment will never happen again.
19. Treat yourself once a week: take time out; have a massage; enjoy a special outing with a loved one.
20. Acknowledge that confidence – like happiness – comes from within and is not dependent on external sources or on other people's approval.

Step 7 – Find your passion in life

If you haven't yet found your passion, finding something outside of work in which you can lose yourself – even for five or ten minutes now and then – can be helpful to avoid over-thinking or over-analysing, which can become a habit in people experiencing anxiety and panic symptoms. By losing yourself, I mean that you don't notice the time passing, as you are so wrapped up in what you are doing. One minute you start doing the activity and the next thing you think is: 'Is that the time? I didn't realise it was so late!' You will know you are on the right track when this occurs.

Generally, activities where you lose track of time are those which require your full concentration. For example, creative activities such as pottery, art, craft, or even learning some new dance steps, where you are so caught up in the moment and there is no time for self-analysis or over-thinking, are all conducive to improving your sense of wellbeing. Ever tried throwing pottery on a wheel? You can be so focused on keeping that piece of clay centred and building it up into a pot that you simply lose track of time. And the best thing is that it doesn't matter if you make a mistake – you can start all over again!

Becoming involved in your community in an area you feel strongly about may also lead to a more fulfilling life.

Self-esteem

Self-esteem and self-confidence go hand in hand. Boosting self-esteem was a popular topic in the 1990s, but nowadays it seems to have gone out of fashion. If your self-esteem has taken a decline due to your health issues, there are several ways to deal with this. Counsellors can take you through some sessions to guide you, which may help you to get back on track. In addition, several books on self-esteem can be found in bookshops and in libraries or you may find a course online.

Improving your confidence and self-esteem may help you to make plans for the future, if you need – or want – to make changes in your life. For further reading on self-esteem, please see the bibliography at the end of this book.

Virtual friends just 'click' – real friends call to see how you are or arrange to meet socially.

Virtual friends are a poor substitute for real friends. Virtual friends just 'click' – real friends call to see how you are or arrange to meet. It's better to concentrate on a few real friends and build a support network rather than relying on virtual friends, although these can be helpful in the short term, particularly if you feel isolated.

Further exercises on the Nose-breathing Pyramid

So far we have talked about nose-breathing while walking (levels 1 and 2 on the Nose-breathing Pyramid). You may also have done a little walking on an incline or climbed stairs while nose-breathing. The initial objective is to walk for thirty minutes while comfortably nose-breathing. Then, when you have mastered thirty minutes of walking while nose-breathing, you are ready to progress to the next levels, if you wish.

You may want to take things further and get back into an exercise routine or play a sport, and this is entirely possible while predominantly nose-breathing, it just takes time and patience.

The next steps on the pyramid may seem quite difficult at first, but with practice you can become very competent.

When you are ready to tackle levels 3 to 7 on the Nose-breathing Pyramid, the following strategies may be introduced *gradually* over the next few weeks. Don't forget to take it step by step, and don't try everything at once or skip ahead to the next level before you are ready. You will know that you are ready when you can comfortably nose-breathe at levels 1 and 2.

It is normal for breathing to deepen or even to be audible when we exercise more vigorously, for example at levels 3 to 7 on the Nose-breathing Pyramid.

- Walk a little more quickly while nose-breathing.
- Walk on an incline or a hill for short periods while nose-breathing.
- Take the stairs – but slow down so you can comfortably nose-breathe.
- Interval training as described last week, until you can jog for twenty minutes while nose-breathing.
- When you are comfortable with levels 1 to 7 on the pyramid you will be ready to try a sport or fitness regimen. Before starting these activities I recommend that you get some professional advice or see a fitness coach.
- Swimming is a great way to improve breathing, but start with the easiest stroke to do while nose-breathing: backstroke. When you are more confident and comfortable, you may try some of the other swimming strokes.

Remember, the Nose-breathing Pyramid is *not* primarily a fitness regimen – although it may coincidentally increase fitness – but is aimed at increasing and retaining carbon dioxide by nose-breathing. Another benefit is the endorphins, the feel-good hormones, which are produced during and following exercise.

Remember to take it slowly; in my experience, most people take three to six weeks to be able to comfortably nose-breathe while jogging or exercising.

However, if fitness and strenuous exercise are not your forte, just continue to move around and improve your breathing pattern through daily activities. Our hunter-gatherer ancestors probably only ran when they had to, e.g. to get out of danger or trap an animal for food, but they would have needed to walk for hours each day in order to find food or shelter.

Ending avoidance

Q.   How do you eat an elephant?
A.   Bit by bit!

In the past, you may have avoided certain places or activities that you associated with anxiety or panic symptoms, and you may have noted these in your diary. If your breathing and posture have sufficiently improved, and you are feeling more confident at dealing with anxiety and panic symptoms, you may feel ready to tackle the avoidance issues or those no-go zones, and stop allowing them to dominate your thinking and your decisions.

When you are ready to confront avoidance issues, you may do this like eating an elephant: bit by bit. (I have seen elephants in the wild in Africa and they are now an endangered species, so I am speaking metaphorically here, of course!) This approach will help you to get back on track and consign the memories of anxiety and panic to where they belong: in the past.

Avoiding situations or events that triggered anxiety or panic attacks in the past form part of the coping mechanisms you developed, and have probably served you well, but perhaps it's time to move on and address the issues that are holding you back.

If you have been severely affected and constrained by your symptoms, you may need some help from a therapist or counsellor, particularly if you don't feel confident about tackling these avoidance issues on your own. However, for many people, just doing small things and gradually taking back control of their lives as their breathing improves may be all that is needed.

Going back to the place where you previously had panic attacks and which you have been avoiding may take a little time and planning. For example, just taking a very short trip to the previously avoided area accompanied by a friend or family member may be enough to boost your confidence and allow for longer visits later, before finally visiting the place alone. You don't have to do it all on your own, and you can build on your successes. Make sure that you know the Controlled Breathing Exercise from Week 1 off by heart, as this will give you more confidence and help you to address the situations you have been avoiding.

Not quite the end

We have come a long way, and although this may be the end of the breathing retraining exercise strategies and techniques, it may not be the end of your breathing retraining program. I recommend that you complete another breathing questionnaire at the end of this week, as this will help you assess your progress to see how you've improved. You may need to continue with the exercises for a further period until you are more comfortable with your breathing pattern, and nose-breathing within the normal range becomes automatic, even in times of stress.

At the end of this week, I recommend that you take time to read the following chapter, which contains some important information about letting go and moving on with your life.

WEEK 4: BREATHING RETRAINING CHECKLIST	
ACTIVITIES	❑ **De-stress and relaxation**: start some easy stress-reducing/relaxation strategies as described this week. ❑ **Nose-breathing Pyramid**: advance through the steps as appropriate for your fitness level. ❑ **Food and nutrition**: continue with the guidelines from last week. ❑ **Stretch**: do your stretches periodically during the day. ❑ **Reading exercise**: continue to do two to three minutes per day, until it feels comfortable. ❑ **Daily diary**: complete before bed every day. ❑ **Avoidance or no-go zones**: if necessary, start to take steps to address the issues discussed this week. ❑ **Breathing questionnaire**: at the end of this week, complete another breathing questionnaire and compare your progress with your baseline level at the start of the program.
BREATHING	❑ At this stage, gentle **nose-breathing** is becoming automatic. Monitor your breathing now and then while in stressful situations or when exercising.
POSTURE	❑ By now your **posture** should be improved but continue to monitor it – particularly in times of stress.
SYMPTOMS	❑ Continue to use the **Controlled Breathing Exercise** or **Short Pause Breathing Exercise** if you experience symptoms.
SLEEP	❑ Continue to **sleep** only on your side.

CHAPTER 21

Moving forward

A sense of healing and tranquillity

Congratulations!

You have made it to the end of your program. By now you are probably sleeping better, feeling better and standing taller, and feel ready to tackle life again. But don't be too concerned if you need to repeat some of the exercises described in this book for longer than four weeks. Four weeks is a very short time, particularly if you have had symptoms for months or even years, or if your symptoms were severe. Everyone heals at a different rate and some people may need more time. So take it at *your* pace – you are in charge here.

Sometimes, increases in stress and the accompanying anxiety and panic symptoms may have led to a sense of feeling overwhelmed. Some of my clients describe this as a kind of inertia: you can't go back, but neither do you feel that you can safely move forwards, and it becomes extremely hard to see a way out. After their breathing retraining course, however, most of my clients are full of ideas on how to move forwards.

Now that your breathing pattern and symptoms have improved, it may be time to take stock and start moving ahead and planning for the future. It's also time to start seeing yourself as someone who *had* a breathing issue – which is now largely eliminated or at least manageable – and to move on and live life to its fullest.

The reality is that life is not perfect;
it is full of compromises.

We sometimes talk about dream homes, dream cars, dream careers, perfect partners or soulmates. But the reality is that life is not perfect; it is full of compromises, and that is what makes it so interesting.

If you think about it, in the western world we are living longer than previous generations, we have greater creature comforts, better standards of living, better education and more abundant food choices than ever before in the history of humankind. But the question is: are we more content or happier than our ancestors?

The fact is that life involves pain, and there is no such thing as perfection. In recent years, programs and books on living in the moment and on mindfulness have become fairly popular. For some people, these may be a helpful reminder of what life is really all about. If you feel you are constantly pursuing goals at the expense of living in the moment, there are courses available on mindfulness, as well as several books. Some of these are listed in the bibliography at the end of this book.

Professor Craig Olsson, researcher in emotional wellbeing, says, 'The key to leading a full and meaningful life is to forget about the pursuit of happiness … A full and meaningful life isn't a life full of happiness. It's a life where the full spectrum of emotions can be encountered and processed in order to grow the individual.'[1] This is a very different and perhaps much more realistic notion than we have been led to believe over the last couple of decades. Dr Russ Harris's book *The Happiness Trap* provides some very good advice on how to stop pursuing happiness, live in the moment and create a more meaningful life.[2]

Making decisions

Being open to new opportunities is great. However, it's best to take things slowly and avoid taking serious risks. Bearing all this in mind, if you *have* been putting your life on hold due to symptoms, it may be time to start planning for your future. You know your situation better than anyone, and you may now be full of ideas.

Wise decisions are practical decisions. For example, it's not wise to quit your job until you have a new one to go to. If you need some professional help, consulting a life coach may be helpful. Or you could try talking to someone who is an expert in the field you have in mind. You don't start out by climbing the highest mountain; you need to practise on smaller mountains first.[3]

Of course, planning does not need to be as significant as changing your career or moving to a new location. You may just need to get back into the swing of things and start enjoying life again. Here are some suggestions:

- Plan to visit a loved one you haven't seen for a while.
- Plan a celebration with your loved one/s when you have completed the four weeks of your breathing retraining program.
- Plan an outing with friends.
- Perhaps take up a hobby or enrol in a class.
- Plan a holiday or perhaps schedule a weekend away.

Feel-good strategies

Have you tried complimenting or going out of your way to help someone recently? Helping others may assist you to regain a sense of connection. One occasion that comes to mind is when I commented on a bank employee's beautiful green eyes (they were indeed beautiful). She was delighted, and she commented that it made her day, and of course it made me feel good too. Just yesterday, I stopped to help an older lady who was trying to wheel her wayward shopping trolley up an incline in the wind and rain, using one hand to steer the trolley while balancing an umbrella in the other hand. It only took a few seconds of my time, but her look of gratitude and her smile were worth far more than those few seconds.

Take time to compliment a loved one for what a great job they do as a wife, husband, mother, father, partner, son or daughter. It will mean more to them than you can imagine.

Perhaps try some of these strategies. You may be surprised by the outcome! Just make sure the compliments are genuine.

- I like your …
- What beautiful eyes!

- That is clever; I wish I could do that!
- What lovely handwriting!
- Show me how you do that ...

Feeling good about yourself through interacting with others will help you to let go and, if needed, help to increase your self-confidence. It's part of our heritage of feeling good and comfortable with our tribe.

If you are symptom-free

After the end of Week 4 (or when you are ready), you might like to consider gradually reducing some of the suggested breathing retraining strategies and activities. Life won't fall apart if you don't always take a daily walk, but by now you will be aware of the need to be careful with your breathing pattern, especially when under stress. Also, you will realise that the need to nose-breathe at all times and to sleep on your side are vitally important, and these need to be continued indefinitely. In any case, these will be almost second-nature by now.

If you are feeling better and no longer having anxiety and panic attacks, you could stop the daily diary at the end of Week 4, but you may want to continue to implement some of the strategies and suggestions we have incorporated over the past few weeks, e.g. de-stressing activities. If you want to move on to fitness, exercise or sports programs then you will need to continue with the advice provided in Week 3 for levels 3 to 8 on the Nose-breathing Pyramid.

Not yet symptom-free?

Not everyone heals at the same pace. It takes time for your new and improved breathing pattern to become automatic, so it's wise to be aware of your breathing and continue to monitor the situation, particularly if you are not yet symptom-free. You may continue with the breathing retraining exercises for a few weeks and then re-assess the situation. If you are still struggling and need further help, you may need to complete a course of breathing retraining with an accredited practitioner. For details, please see Appendix 1.

For those people who need to work on avoidance issues, getting professional help from a therapist may be an option. You will need to continue to ensure that you are gently nose-breathing while you are dealing with stressful situations or events.

Time to let go

For months, years or even decades you may have become accustomed to thinking of yourself as a person whose life is dominated by stress, anxiety and/or panic attacks. But now that you have significantly improved or even eliminated those symptoms – which you now realise were the result of a disordered breathing pattern – you are ready to let go and to start thinking of yourself as healed. We are not defined by our symptoms or conditions, even if they do take over our lives occasionally. We are human beings first, second and last. Once your breathing is improved and your symptoms are reduced or eliminated, it's time to let go.

By now you will most likely be feeling, and looking, a lot better. Many times, I have seen people look younger following their breathing retraining course, as they begin to let go of the burden that stress, anxiety and panic symptoms have imposed on them. And in my classes, people frequently comment that others on the course look years younger! Most people lose that anxious, tired, grey look or pallor they had before they started the breathing retraining course. It's not unusual for women to attend the final session with a new hairdo or hair colour. Their posture is better and they are walking tall, shoulders back, looking more relaxed and confident. In addition, they are sleeping better and have more energy and, best of all, they have that old sparkle back in their eyes!

But letting go isn't easy, and for people who may have begun to think that their symptoms were there for life, it's sometimes one of the hardest things to do. If that is the case, maybe it's time to talk about your experiences with a trusted friend or loved one, or a counsellor. Discussing the issues in this way may help to put things in perspective so that you can clarify issues and start to let go. At the end of breathing retraining courses, I say to my clients, 'You don't need to do breathing exercises for life. There will come a time when all this will seem like a distant memory,' and people visibly relax and start looking forward to the future.

Occasionally I run into former clients in the street and I am struck by how different they look – not just healthier, but happy and relaxed, and full of what the French call joie de vivre. It brings home to me that I see clients at a very vulnerable time in their lives, and it's always a pleasure and a privilege to see how well they look when I meet them later on. I am delighted to hear that many of them have made meaningful changes in their lives, for example, changed their career, moved to a different city, state or even country, or found a significant other, or are just feeling and looking healthier.

They sometimes say, 'You changed my life!' But I don't like to take all the credit for the improvement in their health; I smile and thank them, and then remind them that I just provided the tools – they did the work.

So congratulate yourself and celebrate – you have done all the work!

I hope that you have found within yourself a sense of healing and tranquillity, and I wish you continued good health.

Resources

Anxiety UK Infoline – 03444 775 774
Samaritans – 116 123 Emotional support (free to call from within the UK and Ireland, 24 hours a day)
Mind Infoline – 0300 123 3393 or text 864963

Breathing retraining information

http://www.buteykobayside.com – Mary Birch's website
http://www.buteyko.info – Buteyko Institute of Breathing & Health

Online health information and support

http://www.anxietyuk.org.uk – Support organisation for anxiety, stress, panic and anxiety based depression.
http://www.mind.org.uk – Information on anxiety and panic
http://www.samaritans.org – Information on the Samaritans' support organisation.
http://www.nice.org.uk – National Institute for Health and Care Excellence, information on generalised anxiety disorder and panic disorder.
http://www.nhs.uk – Information on anxiety and panic.

Meditation

www.headspace.com/headspace-meditation-app – Guided
Meditation and Mindfulness – The Headspace App

Mindfulness, stress reduction

http://www.palousemindfulness.com – free online course

The Science of Happiness

https://www.class-central.com/course/edx-the-science-of-
happiness-1781 – Free online course from Berkeley, University of
California

Finding a breathing retraining practitioner

If you decide that you would prefer to do a more formal course with the help of an accredited breathing retraining practitioner, there are a number of considerations to bear in mind. Care is needed in selecting a breathing retraining practitioner, as the breathing retraining methods available may vary considerably. The breathing retraining method I am familiar with and teach is the Buteyko method, which was developed by Russian doctor Professor Konstantin Buteyko. This method advocates normalisation of the breathing pattern. Other breathing retraining methods may differ. Buteyko Institute of Breathing & Health (BIBH) practitioners are trained and regulated according to the standards of the institute; they are required to successfully complete several practical and written assessments before registration. And they are required to practise in accordance with the institute's code of professional conduct. A list of practitioners is provided on the institute's website. If there is no BIBH practitioner listed in your area, it might be worth asking the institute through an email via their website if BIBH practitioners run courses in your area from time to time.

If there are no BIBH practitioners available in your area, there are a number of important questions to ask any potential breathing retraining practitioner before agreeing to enrol with them:

- Which method of breathing retraining does the practitioner use? What is involved? If any mouth-breathing or deep breathing is involved, it is not appropriate.
- Where, and for how long, did the practitioner study breathing retraining?
- Did the practitioner take practical exams or written exams – or both – to obtain a qualification or a credential to teach breathing retraining? Which professional breathing retraining association are they accredited with?
- How long has the practitioner been teaching this method to clients with anxiety and panic?

You may be able to find some of the answers to these questions from the practitioner's website, but personal communication is recommended to confirm their expertise and experience. From their answers you will gain a fair idea of their level of expertise and proficiency. Check with their professional association that they are accredited to practise. Generally, a professional organisation's website will have a list of their accredited practitioners. If they have completed their training in a weekend or two while learning the method and there were no written exams, no practical assessments and no supervised practical experience, that person is probably not the most appropriate person to teach you how to improve your breathing.

Please see the Buteyko Institute of Breathing & Health website: www.buteyko.info

Glossary

Adrenal glands – two glands located on top of the kidneys that produce the stress hormones adrenaline and cortisol.

Adrenaline – the fight-or-flight hormone produced by the adrenal glands.

Agoraphobia – a fear of crowded places.

Alexander Technique – a program aimed at improving posture through the correct use of muscles.

Amygdalae – structures in the brain that form part of the limbic system and are related to memory and emotions, and in particular to fear.

Anxiety – a feeling of emotional discomfort experienced in relation to a perceived stressful event or circumstance, which if prolonged or severe may lead to physical and/or psychological symptoms.

Apnoea – a pause in breathing. See also **Sleep apnoea**.

Assertiveness – a feeling of confidence in negotiating and dealing with life situations, without the need to be aggressive.

Autonomic nervous system – part of the nervous system that regulates unconscious and involuntary responses such as the heart and breathing rates, and is associated with the flight-or-flight and relaxation, or rest-and-digest, responses.

Beta-blockers – a type of medication used in several conditions, including high blood pressure and angina, but also used in anxiety, to control tremor or rapid pulse rates.

BIBH – Buteyko Institute of Breathing & Health, the organisation that regulates and represents practitioner members who teach breathing retraining.

Bohr effect – a phenomenon whereby pH levels in the blood determine effective oxygen release from haemoglobin in our red blood cells. Discovered by Danish scientist Christian Bohr in 1903.

Breathing pattern – how we breathe, in terms of breathing rhythm, regularity, rate, posture and locus of breathing, e.g. diaphragm or upper-chest breathing.

Breathing retraining (may also be known as 'breathing training', 'breathing re-education') – a method of improving the breathing pattern with a specific program of breathing exercises, strategies and techniques.

Bronchial – branches of the bronchus or air tubes in the lungs.

Buteyko breathing techniques – a method of breathing retraining developed by Russian doctor Professor Konstantin Buteyko in the 1950s.

Buteyko Institute Method (BIM) – the method of breathing retraining used by practitioners who are members of a professional organisation called the Buteyko Institute of Breathing & Health (BIBH).

Capnography – continuous measurement of the end-tidal carbon dioxide levels expressed in waveform as opposed to just a number, as in capnometry below.

Capnometer – an instrument used to measure, monitor or assess carbon dioxide levels.

Capnometry – a way of measuring end-tidal carbon dioxide ($ETCO_2$) levels as a person exhales using a scientific instrument called a capnometer. See also **End-tidal carbon dioxide**.

Carbon dioxide (CO_2) – an important gas produced by the body's cells as they produce energy; carbon dioxide levels within the normal range are critical for our survival.

Cardiac output – the amount of blood pumped out by the heart per minute.

Cerebral hypoxia – reduced oxygen to the brain cells.

Cortisol – a naturally occurring hormone produced by the adrenal cortex, which is necessary for everyday living and is increased in times of physical trauma or stress.

CPR – cardio-pulmonary resuscitation, a method that attempts to revive someone who has stopped breathing, or whose heart is not pumping.

Disordered breathing – see **Dysfunctional breathing**.

Dysfunctional breathing – a condition where the breathing pattern is disordered, e.g. due to over-breathing or irregular/erratic breathing.

Dyspnoea – difficulty in breathing.

End-tidal carbon dioxide ($ETCO_2$) – the carbon dioxide level at the end or 'tide' of each exhalation.

Endorphins – feel-good hormones produced naturally in the body in response to a pleasurable experience, e.g. listening to music, or running for prolonged periods.

Fight-or-flight response – a primitive survival response that puts the body on high alert and allows us to fight or flee from a predator or dangerous situation.

Ghrelin – a hormone produced in the stomach that controls appetite.

Glycaemic Index – describes the effect of various foods on blood glucose levels.

Hyperventilation – breathing more air than is required for adequate exchange of gases in the body, i.e. outside of the physiological norm. Also called 'over-breathing'.

Hyperventilation syndrome – a medical condition that involves chronic and severe over-breathing, which may lead to numerous physical and psychological symptoms.

Hypocapnoea – reduced carbon dioxide levels, which may be due to over-breathing or hyperventilation.

Hypoglycaemia – a condition where blood sugar levels fall below the normal range and may lead to symptoms such as headache, sweating, shaking/trembling, spaciness and anxiety.

Hypoxia – a state or condition whereby oxygen levels in the body are reduced.

Insomnia – inability to sleep.

Irritable bowel syndrome (IBS) – a condition diagnosed by a doctor when the patient has experienced a number of bowel issues for several months and where there is no underlying pathology evident.

Leptin – a hormone that is produced in the fat cells and helps us feel full.

Limbic system – a part of the nervous system that plays a pivotal role in behaviour and relates to memory, emotions, fears and survival.

Mediterranean diet – a type of diet traditionally followed in the Mediterranean region, in countries such as Italy and Greece, which emphasises vegetables, fruits, nuts, seeds, seafood, wholegrains, spices, herbs and olive oil.

Melatonin – a naturally occurring hormone produced by the pineal gland that varies during daytime and night-time and helps us to sleep.

Metabolism – the process by which food is broken down and converted to energy.

Microbiome – body ecosystems, e.g. the gut microbiome, which contains trillions of 'good' bacteria, viruses and yeasts, which contribute to our health when kept in balance.

Minute volume – the total air inhaled during one minute of breathing.

Over-breathing – breathing in a greater volume of air than is required for adequate exchange of gases in the body. See also **Hyperventilation**.

Panic attacks – a condition where a person experiences repeated episodes of panic and associated physical and psychological symptoms, sometimes without an obvious cause.

Panic disorder – the medical terminology for a condition where there are repeated panic attacks.

Parasympathetic nervous system – part of the autonomic nervous system, which is related to relaxation or the rest-and-digest response.

Pathology – relating to disease.

pH – a scale used to measure the relative acidity or alkalinity of a solution.

Pineal gland – a tiny gland located in the brain that produces and regulates melatonin.

Residual volume – the amount of air remaining in the lungs after exhalation.

Respiratory alkalosis – a disturbance in acid-base balance due to alveolar hyperventilation, leading to a decrease in the partial

pressure of arterial carbon dioxide. May be due to extreme
anxiety or other medical conditions.

Ruminate – a habit of worrying excessively and thinking about
stressful events or concerns.

Self-esteem – the state of how we feel about situations and events in
relation to our confidence levels.

Sleep apnoea – a condition where a person stops breathing while
asleep due to an obstructed or partially obstructed upper
airway.

Stress – a condition/situation where we experience a physical,
emotional or psychological reaction to challenging life events.
See also **Stressor**.

Stressor – an event or situation that may trigger stress-related
symptoms.

Sympathetic nervous system – part of the nervous system that
allows us to be vigilant and ready to fight or flee.

Syndrome – a collection of signs and/or symptoms which occur in a
medical condition, usually where there is no known pathology
or disease evident.

Tetany – a condition characterised by cramping, spasms and muscle
twitching, and flexion in the ankle and wrist joints. Can be
due to hyperventilation or other medical conditions.

Vasoconstriction – a condition where there is constriction or
narrowing of blood vessels.

Vasomotor – relates to the nerves and muscles that regulate or
control the calibre of blood vessels, thereby altering blood flow,
e.g. narrowing the arteries of the heart in angina, or spasms in
arteries to the brain during panic attacks or other conditions.

Selected bibliography

Agus, D, (2011), *The End of Illness*, Simon & Schuster, New York

Burns, D, (2000), *10 Days to Great Self-Esteem*, Vermilion, London

Caro, J, (2015), *Plain-Speaking Jane: From high anxiety to not giving a toss – a (mostly) fearless memoir*, Pan Macmillan Australia, Sydney

Catlin, G, (1870), *Shut Your Mouth and Save Your Life* (4th ed.), N. Truebner & Co, London

Devi, G, (2012), *A Calm Brain: How to relax into a stress-free, high-powered life*, Plume, New York

Fried, R, (1999), *Breathe Well, Be Well*, John Wiley & Sons Inc, New York

Harris, R, (2007), *The Happiness Trap: Stop Struggling, Start Living*, Exisle Publishing Limited, New South Wales

Harris, R, and Aisbett, B, (2013), *The Happiness Trap Pocketbook: An illustrated guide on how to stop struggling and start living*, Exisle Publishing Limited, New South Wales

Howell, C, and Murphy, M, (2011), *Release Your Worries: A guide to letting go of stress and anxiety*, Exisle Publishing Limited, New South Wales

Kellman, R, (2017), *The Whole Brain Diet: The microbiome solution to heal depression, anxiety, and mental fog without prescription drugs*, Scribe Publications, Melbourne

Meares, A, (1982), *Relief Without Drugs*, Fontana/Collins, Melbourne

Mosley, M, (2017), *The Clever Guts Diet: How to revolutionise your body from the inside out* (ebook), Simon & Schuster, London

Myers, A, (2014), *The Autoimmune Solution* (ebook), HarperCollins, USA

Sapolsky, R M, (2004), *Why Zebras Don't Get Ulcers* (ebook), Henry Holt and Company, New York

Solovitch, S, (2015), *Playing Scared: My journey through stage fright* (ebook), Bloomsbury, USA

Warrell, M, (2015), *Brave: 50 Everyday Acts of Courage to Thrive in Work, Love and Life*, John Wiley & Sons Ltd, Australia

Asthma: breathing retraining publications

Adelola, et al, (2013), 'Role of Buteyko Breathing Technique in asthmatics with nasal symptoms', *Clinical Otolaryngology*, April; 38(2):190–1

Austin, et al, (2009), 'Buteyko Breathing Technique reduces hyperventilation-induced hypocapnoea and dyspnoea after exercise in asthma', *Pulmonary Rehabilitation*, B58 A3409

Borg, et al, (2004), 'The Buteyko Method increases end-tidal CO_2 and decreases ventilatory responsiveness in asthma', The Australian and New Zealand Society of Respiratory Science Ltd. 2004 Annual Scientific Meeting

Bowler, et al, (1998), 'Buteyko breathing techniques in asthma: a blinded randomised controlled trial', *Medical Journal of Australia*, Dec 7–21; 169:11–2.

Burgess, et al, (2011), 'Systematic review of the effectiveness of breathing retraining in asthma management', *Respiratory Medicine*, 5(6) http://informahealthcare.com/doi/abs/10.1586/ers.11.69

Cooper, et al, (2003), 'Effect of two breathing exercises (Buteyko and pranayama) in asthma: a randomised controlled trial', *Thorax*, 58:674–9

Cowie, et al, (2008), 'A randomised controlled trial of the Buteyko technique as an adjunct to conventional management of asthma', *Respiratory Medicine*, May, 102(5):726–32

Hassan, et al, (2012), 'Effect of Buteyko breathing technique on patients with bronchial asthma', *Egyptian Journal of Chest Diseases and Tuberculosis*, 61, pp235–41

Lina, et al, (2014), 'Effectiveness of Buteyko Method in Asthma Control and Quality of Life of School-age Children', academia.edu

McGowan, J, (2003), 'Health Education: Does the Buteyko Institute Method make a difference?' *Thorax*, Vol 58, suppl III, p28

McHugh, et al, (2006), 'Buteyko breathing technique and asthma in children: a case series', *The New Zealand Medical Journal*, May 19, 119(1234)

McHugh, et al, (2003), 'Buteyko Breathing Technique (BBT) for asthma: an effective intervention', *The New Zealand Medical Journal*, Dec 12, 116(1187)

Opat, et al, (2000), 'A clinical trial of the Buteyko Breathing Technique in asthma as taught by a video', *Journal Asthma*, 37(7):557–64

Ravinder, et al, (2012), 'A Study of Effects of Buteyko Breathing Technique on Asthmatic Patients', *Indian Journal of Physiotherapy and Occupational Therapy – An International Journal*, 6(2):224–8

Ruth, A, (2014), 'The Buteyko breathing technique in effective
    asthma management', *Nursing in General Practice*, 7(2):14–16
Villareal, M C, et al, (2014), 'Effect of Buteyko Method on Asthma
    Control and Quality of Life of Filipino Adults with Bronchial
    Asthma', *JMHM* (*The Journal of MacroTrends in Health and
    Medicine*), Vol 2 Issue 1

Sleep apnoea: breathing retraining publications

Birch, M, (2004), 'Obstructive sleep apnoea and breathing
    retraining, clinical update', *Australian Nursing Journal*,
    August, 12(2):27–29
Birch, M, (2012), 'Sleep apnoea: a survey of breathing
    retraining', *Australian Nursing Journal*, October, 20(4):40–1,
    www.buteyko.info
Birch, M, (2012), 'Sleep apnoea and breathing retraining. To what
    extent is the Buteyko Institute Method of breathing retraining
    effective for sleep apnoea? A survey of Buteyko Institute
    practitioners' experiences with clients suffering from sleep
    apnoea,' www.buteyko.info
Graham, T, (2012), *Relief from Snoring and Sleep Apnoea*, Penguin,
    Australia

Acknowledgements

I owe my heartfelt thanks to a great number of people who encouraged and supported me, and inspired me to write this book.

In particular, I would like to thank my husband, my children and my family and friends for their continued love and support since I first started this book in 2014.

To my Buteyko trainer and mentor, Paul O'Connell, CEO of the Buteyko Institute of Breathing & Health, I owe a debt of gratitude and thanks for his integrity and his willingness to help and support me in all matters related to breathing retraining over the years since I first encountered the Buteyko Method in 1998. I would also like to thank Paul for his insightful comments on an earlier draft of *Breathe*. Also, I owe special thanks to practitioner members of the Buteyko Institute of Breathing & Health who generously shared their knowledge and expertise in a collegial way through an online forum and at seminars and conferences.

My thanks also go to the teams at Hachette Australia and Little, Brown Book Group, UK, for their professional and helpful approach in preparing the book for publication and making *Breathe* a reality.

Last, but by no means least, I would like to thank my clients who encouraged me to write this book and without whom it would never have been possible. I am forever grateful. You have taught me more about life, endurance and breathing than I could ever find in books.

Endnotes

Introduction

1   Interview with K P Buteyko, taken in 1982, (1990), *The Buteyko Method: An Experience of Use in Medicine*, Patriot Publishers, Moscow

2   Birch, M, (2015), 'Breathing Retraining in Anxiety and Panic Disorder', *Australian Nursing and Midwifery Journal*, 23(4):31–3, PMID 26665642

Chapter 1

1   www.mind.org.uk; See also: Mental health and wellbeing in England, Adult Psychiatric Morbidity Survey 2014, The National Archives.

2   See for example: Lum, L C, (1975), 'Hyperventilation: the tip and the iceberg', *Journal of Psychosomatic Research*, Pergamon Press, 19:375–83; Fried, R, (1999), *Breathe Well, Be Well*, John Wiley & Sons Inc, New York; Liotti, M, et al, (2002), 'Neural Correlates of CO_2-induced air hunger in high and low trait-anxiety volunteers', NeuroImage Human Brain Mapping 2002 Meeting, *Elsevier Science (USA)*; Meuret, A E, and Ritz, T, (2010), 'Hyperventilation in Panic Disorder and Asthma: Empirical Evidence and Clinical Strategies', *Int J Psychophysiol*, 78(1): 68–79, published online May 2010, PMID 20685222

3   The instrument I use, called the CapnoTrainer® (Better Physiology), is an educational instrument designed for enhancing performance through learning and teaching good breathing behaviour. It is not intended for medical diagnosis or treatment

4   Van den Hout, M A, Hoekstra, R, Arntz, A, Christiaanse, M,
       Ranschaert, W, and Schouten, E, (1992), 'Hyperventilation is not
       diagnostically specific to panic patients', *Psychosomatic Medicine*,
       54(2):182–91, Pub Med 1565755

Chapter 2
1   Dratcu, L, (2000), 'Panic, hyperventilation and perpetuation
       of anxiety', *Progress Neuropsychopharmacol Biological Psychiatry*,
       24(7):1069–89, PreMedline Identifier: 11131173; Meuret and Ritz,
       op. cit.; Lum, op. cit.

Chapter 3
1   Meuret and Ritz, op. cit.
2   Hegel, M T, and Ferguson, R J, (1996), 'Psychophysiological
       assessment of respiratory function in panic disorder: Evidence for a
       hyperventilation subtype', *Psychosomatic Medicine*, 59(3):224–30
3   Martinez, J M, Kent, J M, Coplan, J D, Brown, S T, Papp, L A,
       Sullivan, G M, Kleber, M, Perepletchikova, F, Fyer, A J, Klein,
       D F, and Gorman, J M, (2001), 'Respiratory Variability in Panic
       Disorder', *Depression and Anxiety*, 14(4):232–7
4   Yates, W R, (2016), 'Anxiety Disorders', www.emedicine.medscape.
       com, article 286227, accessed June 2016
5   Dratcu, op. cit.
6   Meuret and Ritz, op. cit.; Fried, op. cit.; Lum, op. cit.
7   Klein, D F, (1993), 'False suffocation alarms, spontaneous panics,
       and related conditions: an integrative hypothesis', *Archives of General
       Psychiatry*, 50:306–17, Pub Med 8466392
8   The autonomic nervous system is not a separate nervous system. See:
       Tortora, G J, and Anagnostakos, N P, (1987), *Principles of Anatomy
       and Physiology*, (5th ed.), Harper and Row, New York
9   Laffey, J G, and Kavanagh, B P, (2002), 'Hypocapnia', *New England
       Journal of Medicine*, 347(1):43–53
10   Lum, op. cit.
11   Pfortmueller, C A, Pauchard-Neuwerth, S E, Leichte, A B,
       Fiedler, G M, Exadaktylos, A K, and Lindner, G, (2015), 'Primary
       hyperventilation in the emergency department: a first overview',
       PLOS One, 10(6) e0129562
12   Barloon, T J, and Noyes, R, Jr, (1997), 'Charles Darwin and panic
       disorder', *JAMA*, Jan 8; 227(2):138–41, PMID 8990339

13   University of Cambridge, Darwin Correspondence Project, Six things Darwin never said, www.darwinproject.ac.uk

14   Adrenaline was purified in 1901. See: www.serious-science.org/adrenaline-7601

15   See: www.betterhealth.vic.gov.au/health/conditionsandtreatments/panic-attack

Chapter 4

1   Thomas, M, McKinley, R K, Freeman, E, Foy, C, and Price, D, (2004), 'The prevalence of dysfunctional breathing in adults in the community with and without asthma', *Primary Care Respiratory Journal*, 14:78–82. Doi:101016/j.pcrj.2002.10.007

2   The review analysed dysfunctional breathing and hyperventilation syndrome (DB/HVS). Jones, M, Harvey, A, Marston, L, and O'Connell, N E, (2013), 'Breathing exercises for dysfunctional breathing/hyperventilation syndrome in adults', *Cochrane Database of Systematic Reviews*, Issue 5. Art. No.: CD009041. DOI: 10.1002/14651858.CD009041.pub2

3   Profiles of Health Australia, (2012), 'Asthma', *Australian Bureau of Statistics*, 2011–12

4   Fried, op. cit., p45

5   Fried, op. cit., pp164–70

6   Kern, B, (2014), 'Hyperventilation Syndrome', http://emedicine.medscape.com/article/807277-overview, updated September 4, 2014, accessed June 2015

7   Magarian, G J, Middaugh, D A, and Linz, D H, (1983), 'Hyperventilation syndrome: A diagnosis begging for recognition (Topics in Primary Care Medicine)', *Western Journal of Medicine*, May, 138:733–6

8   Jones, et al, op. cit.

9   Evans, R W, (2005), 'Unilateral Paresthesias due to Hyperventilation Syndrome', *Practical Neurology*, Expert Opinion, on-line: researchgate.net; see also: Fried, op. cit., p46

10   This list of potential signs and symptoms was compiled from several sources. See for example: Lewis, B I, (1957), in Fried, R, (1990), *The Breath Connection*, Plenum Press, New York; Fried, 1999; Laffey, op cit; Jones, et al, op. cit. and Kern, op. cit.

11   Jones, et al, op. cit.

12   Fried, op. cit., p53

13   Magarian, et al, op. cit.
14   www.mayoclinic.org
15   Smitherman, T A, Kolivas, E D, and Bailey, J R, (2013), 'Panic disorder and migraine: comorbidity, mechanisms, and clinical implications', *Headache: The Journal of Head and Face Pain*, 53:23–45
16   Martin, V T, Fanning, K M, Serrano, D, Buse, D C, Reed, M L, and Lipton, R B, (2016), 'Asthma is a risk factor for new onset chronic migraine: Results from the American migraine prevalence and prevention study', *Headache: The Journal of Head and Face Pain*, 56:118–31
17   Merikangas, K, (2013), 'Contributions of Epidemiology to our Understanding of Migraine', *Headache*, 53(2):230–46
18   Kern, op. cit.
19   ibid.
20   From a total of 496 records, 495 were excluded because they did not meet the inclusion criteria. Jones et al, op. cit.
21   While the Buteyko method is mentioned in the review, the clinical trial cited was conducted for asthma – not for HVS

Chapter 5
1   The Nijmegen Questionnaire is freely available online. See also: Van Dixhoorn, J, and Folgering, H, (2015), 'The Nijmegen Questionnaire and dysfunctional breathing', *ERJ Open Research*, May; 1(1): 00001-2015

Chapter 6
1   Bowler, S D, Green, A, and Mitchell, C A, (1998), 'Buteyko breathing techniques in asthma: a blinded randomised controlled trial', *The Medical Journal of Australia*, 169(11–12):575–8
2   Tortora and Anagnostakos, op. cit.

Chapter 7
1   Interview with K P Buteyko, 1990
2   ibid.
3   Stalmatski, A, (1997), *Freedom from Asthma: Buteyko's Revolutionary Treatment*, Kyle Cathie Ltd, London
4   Buteiko [sic], K P, (1994), Author's preface to *Buteiko's Method, Method of Volitional Control of Deep Breathing Guide for Training*, Voskresensk, 1994

5   ibid.

6   ibid.

7   Stalmatski, op. cit.

8   Lum, op. cit.

9   ibid.

10   Fried, op. cit., p45

11   Fried, op. cit., p42

Chapter 8

1   Carlin, G, (1870), *Shut Your Mouth and Save Your Life*, (4th ed.), N. Truebner & Co, London

2   Foster, J A, Rinaman, L, and Cryan, J F, (2017), 'Stress & the gut–brain axis: Regulation by the microbiome', *Neurobiology of Stress 7*, (2017) 7, 124–6

3   Evrensel, A, and Ceylan, M E, (2015), 'The Gut–Brain Axis: The Missing Link in Depression', *Clinical Psychopharmacology and Neuroscience*, Dec. 13(3):239–44

4   Rea, K, Dinan, T G, and Cryan, J F, (2016), 'The microbiome: A key regulator of stress and neuroinflammation', *Neurobiology of Stress*, Vol. 4, October 2016, 23–33

5   See: www.hopkinsmedicine.org/health/healthy_aging/healthy_body/the-brain-gut-connection. Accessed March, 2018

6   By the end of 2017 more than 650 scientific papers on the human microbiome had been published. See: www.commonfund.nih.gov/hmp. Accessed March, 2018

7   Opie, et al, (2017), 'A modified Mediterranean dietary intervention for adults with major depression: Dietary protocol and feasibility data from the SMILES trial', *Nutritional Neuroscience*, April 19, PMID 28424045

8   Foster, et al, op. cit.

9   Pirbaglou, et al, (2016), 'Probiotic supplementation can positively affect anxiety and depressive symptoms: a systematic review of randomized controlled trials', *Nutritional Research*, 36(9):889–98, PMID 27632908

10   McKean, J, Naug, H, Nikbakht, E, Amiet, B, and Colson, N, (2017), 'Probiotics and Subclinical Psychological Symptoms in Healthy Participants: A Systematic Review and Meta-Analysis', *Journal of Alternative and Complementary Medicine*, April 23(4): 249–58, PMED ID 27841940

11   See: www.betterhealth.vic.gov.au/health/ConditionsAndTreatments/
        irritable-bowel-syndrome-ibs
12   Sugaya, et al, (2013), 'Irritable bowel syndrome, its cognition,
        anxiety sensitivity, and anticipatory anxiety in panic disorder
        patients', *Psychiatry and Clinical Neurosciences*, 67(6):397–404

Chapter 9
1   Reduced vitamin D levels (from decreased exposure to sunlight)
        may be associated with altered mood and wellbeing
2   Devi, G, (2012), *A Calm Brain: How to relax into a stress-free,
        high-powered life*, Plume, New York
3   ibid.
4   Myers, A, (2014), *The Autoimmune Solution*, (epub ed.), Harper
        Collins, USA
5   Tortora and Anagnostakos, op. cit.
6   Ernst, G, (2017), 'Hidden Signals – The History and Methods
        of Heart Rate Variability', *Frontiers in Public Health*, 5:265,
        doi:103389/pubh.2017.00265
7   Devi, op. cit.
8   Litchfield, P M, (2003), 'A brief overview of the chemistry of
        respiration and the breathing heart wave', *California Biofeedback*,
        Vol. 19 No. 1.
9   Rajmohan, V, and Mohandas, E, (2007), 'The limbic system', *Indian
        Journal of Psychiatry*, Apr–Jun; 49(2):132–9
10   Devi, op. cit.
11   Solovitch, S, (2015), *Playing Scared: My journey through stage fright*,
        (ebook), Bloomsbury, London

Chapter 10
1   Tortora and Anagnostakos, op. cit.
2   Laffey, op. cit.
3   Seddon, K, Morris, K, Baily, J, Potokar, J, Rich, A, Wilson, S,
        Bettica, P, and Nutt, D J, (2011), 'Effects of 7.5% CO_2 challenge
        in generalized anxiety disorder', *Journal of Psychopharmacology*,
        25(1):43–51

Chapter 11
1   Freeman, et al, (2017), 'The effects of improving sleep on mental
        health (OASIS): a randomised controlled trial with mediation

analysis', *Lancet Psychiatry*, 4:749–58; 'Want to Improve Patients' Mental Health? Start with their Sleep', *Medscape*, March 7, 2018

2   *Harvard Mental Health Letter*, July, 2009, 'Sleep and Mental Health', www.health.harvard.edu/newsletter_article/Sleep-and-mental-health, accessed February, 2018

3   Liu, A, Kushida, C A, and Reaven, G M, (2013), 'Habitual shortened sleep and insulin resistance: an independent relationship in obese individuals', *Metabolism*, 62(11):1553–6, PubMed ID 23849514

4   Alnaji, A, Law, G R, and Scott, E M, (2016), 'The role of sleep duration in diabetes and glucose control', (epub ahead of print), *Proceedings of the Nutrition Society*, PubMed ID 27334543

5   See for example: *Harvard Mental Health Letter*, July 2009; www.nhs.uk/Livewell/tiredness-and-fatigue/Pages/lack-of-sleep-health-risks.aspx.

6   Cedernaes, J, Osler, M E, Voisin, S, Brokman, J, Vogel, H, Dickson, S L, Zierath, J R, Schioth, H B, and Benedict, C, (2015), 'Acute Sleep Loss Induces Tissue-Specific Epigenetic and Transcriptional Alteration to Circadian Clock Genes in Men', *The Journal of Clinical Endocrinology and Metabolism*, DOI http://dx.doi.org/10.1210/JC.2015–2284

7   Hegarty, S, (2012), 'The myth of the eight-hour sleep', *BBC World Service News Magazine* online, 22 February, 2012

8   Changa, A, Aeschbacha, D, Duffy, J F, and Czeislera, C A, (2016), 'Evening use of light-emitting eReaders negatively affects sleep, circadian timing, and next-morning alertness', *PNAS*, 112:1232–7

9   Gronli, J, Kristiansen, B, Bjorvatn, B, Nodtvedt, O, Harre, B, and Pallesen, S, (2016), 'Reading from an iPad or from a book in bed: the impact on human sleep. A randomized controlled crossover trial', *Sleep*, DOI: http://dx.doi.org/10.1016/j.sleep.2016.02.006

10   Anderson, P, (2016), 'Excess Street Lighting Affects Sleep', Coverage from the American Academy of Neurology (AAN), March 11, 2016 Annual Meeting, *Medscape Medical News* online report

11   Henry Ford Health System, (2013), 'Don't ignore the snore: Snoring may be early sign of future health risks', *ScienceDaily*, 24 January, www.sciencedaily.com/releases/2013/01/1301241212741.htm

12   Weaver, T E, and Sawyer, A N, (2010), 'Adherence to Continuous Airway Pressure Treatment for Obstructive Sleep Apnea: Implications for Future Interventions', *Indian Journal of Medical Research*, February, 131: 245–258, p1

13   Birch, M, (2012a), 'Sleep Apnoea and Breathing Retraining',
      www.buteyko.info

14   Birch, M, (2012b), 'Clinical Update: Sleep Apnoea – A survey of
      Breathing Retraining', *Australian Nursing Journal*, 20(4):40–41.
      PMID 2325114, www.buteyko.info

15   Birch, M, (2004), 'Obstructive Sleep Apnoea and Breathing
      Retraining, Clinical Update', *Australian Nursing Journal*. August,
      12(2):27–29. PMID 19160562, www.buteyko.info

16   Graham, T, (2012), *Relief from Snoring and Sleep Apnoea*, Penguin,
      Australia

17   Brauser, D, (2016), '"Striking" Link Between Sleep Disturbances
      and Stroke', *Medscape*, August 04

18   Brooks, M, (2017), 'Sleep-Disordered Breathing Raises Risk for
      Cognitive Decline', *Medscape*, August 29

19   Pillar, G, and Shehadeh, N, (2009), 'Abdominal fat and sleep apnea:
      the chicken or the egg?', *Diabetes Care*, February 31, Suppl.2:S303–9

20   Oltmanns, K M, Gehring, H, Rudolf, S, Schultes, B, Schweiger,
      U, Born, J, Fehm, H L, and Peters, A, (2006), 'Persistent
      suppression of resting energy expenditure after acute hypoxia',
      Metabolism, May; 55(5):669–75

21   Taheri, S, Lin, L, Austin, D, Young, T, and Mignot, E, (2004),
      'Short Sleep Duration is Associated with Reduced Leptin, Elevated
      Ghrelin and Increased Body Mass Index', *PLoS Medicine*, 1(3); e62

22   Tschop, M, Weyer, C, Tataranni, P A, Devanarayan, V, Ravussin,
      E, and Heiman, M L, (2001), 'Circulating Ghrelin Levels Are
      Decreased in Human Obesity', *Diabetes*, Vol. 50, April

Chapter 12
1   The amygdalae form part of the limbic system, which evolved in
      early mammals, and record our bad or fearful experiences and other
      emotions
2   McLaren, S, (2004), *Don't Panic: You can overcome anxiety without
      drugs*, Scribe Publications, Melbourne

Chapter 13
1   See: www.cochrane.org
2   Jones, et al, op. cit.
3   ibid.
4   Birch, 2012a, Birch, 2012b; see also: www.buteyko.info

5   *Asthma, anxiety & depression*, joint factsheet, Asthma Australia/ Beyond Blue, 2013

6   Bowler et al, op. cit.

7   ibid.

8   Borg, et al, (2004), 'The Buteyko Method increases end-tidal CO_2 and decreases ventilatory responsiveness in asthma', *The Australian and New Zealand Society of Respiratory Science Ltd. 2004 Annual Scientific Meeting*

9   Austin, et al, (2009), 'Buteyko breathing technique reduces hyperventilation-induced hypocapnoea and dyspnoea after exercise in asthma', *Pulmonary Rehabilitation*, B58 A3409

10   Ravinder, et al, (2012), 'A study of Effects of Buteyko Breathing Technique on Asthmatic Patients', *Indian Journal of Physiotherapy and Occupational Therapy – An International Journal* 6(2):224–8

11   Hassan, et al, (2012), 'Effect of Buteyko breathing technique on patients with bronchial asthma', *Egyptian Journal of Chest Diseases and Tuberculosis*, 61:235–41

12   *Harvard Mental Health Letter*, 2009

Chapter 14

1   The CapnoTrainer®. This instrument is used for educational capnography and is not intended for medical diagnosis or treatment

Chapter 15

1   Interview with Buteyko taken in 1982, op. cit.

Chapter 16

1   Kern, op. cit.

2   Martinez, et al, op. cit.

Chapter 17

1   Nair, et al, (2015), 'Do slumped and upright postures affect stress response? A randomized trial', *Health Psychology*, 34(6), June, http://dx.doi.org/10.1037/hea0000146

Chapter 18

1   St-Onge, M P, Roberts, A, Shechter, A, and Choudhury, A R, (2016), 'Fiber and saturated fat are associated with sleep arousals and slow wave sleep', *Journal of Clinical Sleep Medicine*, 12(1):19–24

2   www.health.harvard.edu/sleep/8-secrets-to-a-good-nights-sleep
3   Bratman, G N, Hamilton, J P, Hahn, K S, Daily, G C, and Gross,
         J J, (2015), 'Nature experience reduces rumination and subgenual
         prefrontal cortex activation', *PNAS*, 112(28):8567–72.
4   Bratman, et al, op. cit.

Chapter 19
2   Frellick, M, (2017), 'Higher coffee intake tied to lower mortality
         risk', *Medscape*, July

Chapter 21
1   Olsson, C, (2015), 'The failed pursuit of happiness', quoted in *dKin*,
         Deakin University Alumni Magazine, Issue 3, p40
2   Harris, R, (2007), *The Happiness Trap: Stop Struggling, Start Living*,
         Exisle Publishing Limited, New South Wales
3   Warrell, M, (2015), *Brave: 50 Everyday Acts of Courage to Thrive in
         Work, Love and Life*, John Wiley & Sons Ltd, Australia

After training as a nurse at Central Middlesex Hospital in London, Mary Birch worked in Australia, the UK and Zambia. Mary also worked as a nurse lecturer and clinical teacher for ten years in Australia. Mary has published several articles on breathing retraining and presents regularly on this topic to healthcare professionals and community groups. Since starting her Melbourne breathing retraining practice in 1999, she has successfully helped numerous clients experiencing stress, anxiety and panic to improve their breathing pattern and transform their lives.

Mary lives in Melbourne with her husband.